A Color Handbo

Skin Diseases in the Elderly

Colby C. Evans, MD

Evans Dermatology Partners
Austin, Texas, USA

Whitney A. High, MD, JD, MEng

Associate Professor, Dermatology and Pathology
Attending, Denver STD and HIV Prevention Clinic
University of Colorado School of Medicine
Denver, Colorado, USA

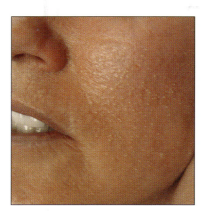

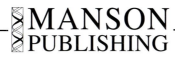

MANSON
PUBLISHING

This book is dedicated to Sara, Quinn, and Malcolm Evans,
whose love and support make everything I do possible.
CE

Dedicated to my M&M's - Misha and Madison.
WH

Image Credits:
St John's Institute of Dermatology – 40, 88, 92, 93, 94, 95, 96, 97, 101, 108, 160, 194, 201, 202, 211, 212, 219, 229, 230; Manson Publishing – 46; Stephen Houston MD –133, 134, 135; Dr Shahid Chaudhry – 213, 214; McGraw Hill – 216, 217.

Copyright © 2012 Manson Publishing Ltd
ISBN: 978-1-84076-154-2

For full details of all Manson Publishing Ltd titles please write to:
Manson Publishing Ltd, 73 Corringham Road, London NW11 7DL, UK.
Tel: +44(0)20 8905 5150
Fax: +44(0)20 8201 9233
Email: manson@mansonpublishing.com
Website: www.mansonpublishing.com

Commissioning editor: Jill Northcott
Project manager: Julie Bennett
Copy editor: Julie Pickard
Layout: DiacriTech, India
Colour reproduction: Tenon & Polert Colour Scanning Ltd, HK
Printed by: New Era Printing Co Ltd, HK

CONTENTS

PART 4
Infestations and infections

Parasitic

Viral

Bacterial

Fungal

PART 5
Metabolic and nutritional disease

PART 6
Skin signs of systemic disease

PREFACE

Geriatric dermatology and geriatric medicine in general will grow exponentially in importance during the coming years. As the average age throughout the Western world rises steadily, and life expectancies lengthen, more and more elderly patients will seek care for a variety of skin conditions.

Certainly some of these skin conditions are particular to, or at least more common in, elderly persons. Other conditions may present at any age, but may represent diagnostic and therapeutic challenges in the aged patient. As the number of elderly patients rises, these challenges will become increasingly common for both the primary care physician and the dermatologist.

Demographic data tell a concise story regarding the population of most Western countries – it is aging quickly. The United States Administration on Aging reports the number of persons >65 years of age will more than double to 71.5 million by 2030. In 2000, persons >65 years of age represented just 12.4% of the total population, but this group will represent at least 20% of the population by 2030.

Similar findings were reported by the United Kingdom Office for National Statistics. In 2006, the fastest-growing segment of the population in the United Kingdom was those persons aged 85 years old and older, with a record-setting 1.2 million people in this category. From 1971 to 2006, the overall population grew 8% while the population of persons >65 grew 31%.

Both the United States and United Kingdom experienced 'baby booms' in the years following World War II. Large spikes in the birth rate at that time have led to large numbers of people now preparing to enter elderly age. Advances in health care and increases in the average lifespan have worked also to increase the numbers further.

These trends foretell enormous change in the practice of medicine. The mix of elderly patients in the practice of the average physician will surely increase. The number of very elderly patients will also rise, potentially straining resources for geriatricians and long-term care facilities.

In dermatology, several trends will result as these changes occur. While skin cancer can occur at any age, most forms are decidedly more common after a lifetime of sun exposure. Non-melanoma skin cancer, in particular basal cell carcinoma and squamous cell carcinoma, will become more prevalent. As the aging process also hinders the retention of moisture in the skin, conditions exacerbated by dry skin (such as psoriasis and eczema) may worsen. As patients age, they also tend to accumulate more benign skin lesions (such as seborrheic keratoses or sebaceous hyperplasia). These benign lesions may lead to irritated examples that require treatment and will need to be differentiated from more concerning lesions.

Treatment can also be more challenging in elderly patients. Older patients tend to take more medications, leading to the increased potential for drug interactions. They may also have age- or disease-related decreases in liver or kidney function and, therefore, have difficulty processing the drugs. Topical therapies can also be more difficult to apply in the setting of arthritis or visual decline.

The purpose of this text is to discuss those dermatologic conditions that occur in the elderly patient. Its goal is not only to help the practitioner diagnose and treat conditions in geriatric dermatology, but to also help target testing and therapy so that it is most useful in this special and rapidly growing patient population.

ABBREVIATIONS

ABCD criteria	asymmetry, border irregularity, color variation, and diameter >6mm
AIDS	acquired immune deficiency syndrome
ANA	antinuclear antibody
AST	aspartate aminotransferase
BSA	body surface area
CA-MRSA	community-acquired methicillin-resistant *Staphylococcus aureus*
CBC	complete blood count
CK	creatine kinase
CT	computed tomography (scan)
ELISA	enzyme-linked immunosorbent assay
ENA	extractable nuclear antigen
ESR	erythrocyte sedimentation rate
HHV	human herpesvirus
HIV	human immunodeficiency virus
HPV	human papillomavirus
HTLV	human T-cell lymphotropic virus
ICU	intensive care unit
Ig	immunoglobulin
IVIG	intravenous immunoglobulin
KOH	potassium hydroxide
KTP	potassium–titanyl–phosphate (laser)
LDH	lactate dehydrogenase
LDL	low-density lipoprotein
MED	minimal erythema dose
MRI	magnetic resonance imaging
MRSA	methicillin-resistant *Staphylococcus aureus*
Nd:YAG	neodymium-doped:yttrium–aluminum–garnet (laser)
NSAID	non-steroidal anti-inflammatory drug
PCR	polymerase chain reaction
PET	positron emission tomography (scan)
PUVA	(oral) psoralen plus ultraviolet A
SSKI	supersaturated potassium iodide
TMP/SMX	trimethoprim/sulfamethoxazole (co-trimoxazole)
UV	ultraviolet

SUGGESTED READING

Bolognia JL, Jorizzo JL, Rapini RP. *Dermatology*. New York: Mosby, 2007.

Burns T, Breathnach S, Cox N, Griffiths C (eds). *Rook's Textbook of Dermatology*. Oxford: Wiley-Blackwell, 2010.

Habif TP. *Clinical Dermatology: A Color Guide to Diagnosis and Therapy*. London: Mosby, 2003.

Rietschel RL., Fowler JF. *Fisher's Contact Dermatitis*, 6th edn. PMPH-USA, 2007.

Wolff K, Goldsmith LA, Katz SI, Gilchrest BA, Paller A, Leffell DJ (eds). *Fitzpatrick's Dermatology in General Medicine*. New York: McGraw-Hill Professional, 2007.

Wolverton SE. *Dermatologic Drug Therapy*. Philadelphia: WB Saunders, 2007.

www.emedicine.medscape.com

www.dermis.net/dermisroot/en/home/index.htm

PART 1

Skin changes with aging

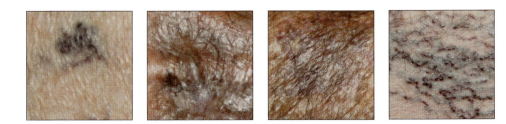

Although elderly patients are prone to a number of skin diseases, there exist also typical age-related skin changes that are not disease associated. Although these changes occur to all patients, should they live long enough, they can have profound effects on the proper function of the skin, and, hence, the patient's corresponding quality of life.

Age-related atrophy

Skin atrophy is commonly seen in elderly patients, evidenced by thinning or fine wrinkling, easy tearing, and bruising. In sun-protected sites, this atrophy usually results in fine, 'cigarette paper' wrinkling of the skin (**1 & 2**). The skin is often light in color compared with chronically sun-exposed skin.

Fat loss, especially on the face and hands (**3**), is quite common with age. Since the fat layer provides a cushion for blood vessels, they become more visible with time and more prone to bleeding with minor trauma. Fat loss, especially in the face and hands, is also a common cosmetic concern for older patients.

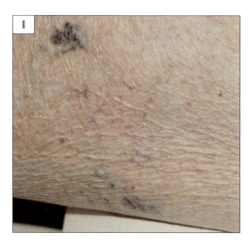

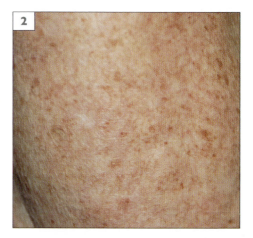

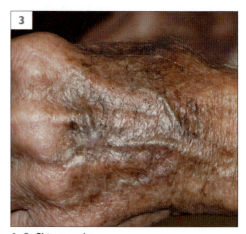

I–3 Skin atrophy.

Solar atrophy

Atrophy is also common on the sun-exposed skin, but in a different form. Solar atrophy often exhibits hyperpigmentation, deep wrinkles, and a 'leathery' appearance. It is commonly seen on the face, neck, forearms, and dorsal hands. It not only leads to easy tearing and bruising of the skin (**4**), but is a sign of chronic sun damage which can lead to other problems, especially skin cancer.

Bruising

Elderly patients often complain of easy bruising and tearing of the skin that leads to bleeding (**4 & 5**). One contributory cause is the blood-thinning medications often taken by elderly patients to prevent myocardial infarction or stroke. Aspirin, warfarin, and clopidogrel are common examples. Other medications, especially NSAIDs, may also increase this tendency. Even patients who do not take such medications, however, may also experience easy bruising due to fat loss and skin atrophy, with subsequent loss of the surrounding supportive collagen near vessels, leading to bruising on the frequently traumatized forearms and hands.

4, 5 Bruising.

Xerosis

As the skin ages, its ability to produce and maintain the normal oils and fats that help retain moisture erodes. The skin becomes drier and moisturizer must be applied more often to avoid itchy, painful, or fissuring skin (**6** see also **84**). Xerosis (skin dryness) is usually worse in the winter due to low humidity and indoor heat. Xerosis may be a problem unto itself or it may worsen common skin conditions such as eczema or psoriasis. It can be particularly difficult for elderly patients to avoid, as bathing and applying moisturizer may be more difficult due to arthritis, visual problems, or other comorbid conditions.

Varicosities

Since gravity attempts to pull all blood towards the feet, the vessels of the legs are under constant pressure. A system of muscular milking and valves helps return the blood to the heart, but these vessels weaken over years of time and pressure, and varicosities are the result. Superficial or deep, red, blue, or purple serpiginous veins are visible on the legs (**7–10**). Varicosities may be both medically and cosmetically troublesome. If they are painful, examination by ultrasound may be necessary followed by vein stripping or endovascular procedures performed with a heat probe or laser. Cosmetically bothersome veins can often be treated with sclerotherapy, the injection of a sclerosant material into the vein causing it to seal closed.

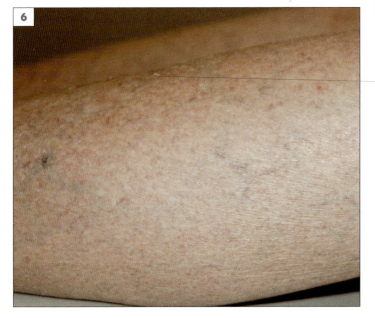

6 Xerosis.

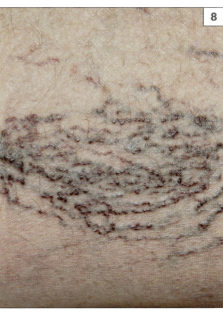

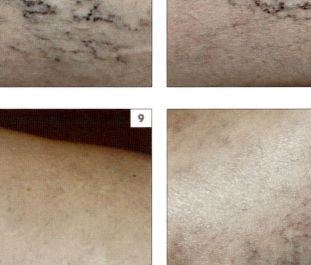

7–10 Varicosities.

PART 2

Inflammatory skin disease

- **Autoimmune**

- **Neutrophilic dermatoses**

- **Allergic and hypersensitivity processes**

- **Photorelated conditions**

- **Other inflammatory conditions**

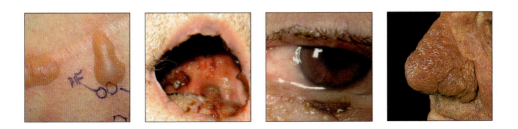

AUTOIMMUNE

Bullous pemphigoid

DEFINITION AND CLINICAL FEATURES

Bullous pemphigoid (BP) is an autoimmune blistering disorder that often results in large, tense, bullae (**11**). These bullae, being subepidermal in origin, are often resistant to rupture and, in comparison to pemphigus, intact blisters on clinical exam are not unexpected. Lesions of BP often appear first on the flexural aspects of the limbs (**12**), including the axilla (**13**). The trunk may be involved as well (**14**). Associated pruritus can be intense.

The face and scalp are not often involved in BP, and while the mucosa may be involved in up to 10–25% of cases, in direct contrast to pemphigus vulgaris, the mucosa is not typically the site of first involvement in this disease. Urticarial BP is a variant that presents with intense itching and erythematous skin lesions, but lacks frank bullae (**15**). Sometimes patients with urticarial BP may never develop blisters and, on occasion, the condition may be present for years before the diagnosis is established.

EPIDEMIOLOGY

BP is chiefly a disease of the elderly. The average age at onset is about 65 years. Females and males are equally affected and the disease is seen in all races. It is not uncommon for a patient with BP to have multiple comorbidities; a factor that must be considered in prescribing treatment with corticosteroids or immunosuppressive medications.

DIFFERENTIAL DIAGNOSIS AND INVESTIGATIONS

Other bullous skin diseases, such as pemphigus, cicatricial pemphigoid, bullous lupus erythematosus, epidermolysis bullosa acquisita, and porphyria cutanea tarda must be considered. Some medications may cause drug-induced bullous disorder resembling BP.

The diagnosis of BP is most easily established by histological analysis. Light microscopy should be performed from the edge of a blister and direct immunofluorescence studies should be performed on normal-appearing perilesional skin (**11**). Routine histology demonstrates a subepidermal vesiculatory process, often with a preponderance of eosinophils in the blister cavity.

Direct immunofluorescence studies demonstrate the deposition of immunoreactants as a band at the dermoepidermal junction of the skin. This pattern of deposition is not specific for BP and it may be seen in cicatricial pemphigoid and epidermolysis bullosa acquisita, as well. Clinical information, the findings of light microscopy, performance of direct immunofluorescence on salt-split skin (with induced separation at the dermoepidermal junction) or indirect immunofluorescence studies using the patient's serum and normal salt-split skin can be used to further refine the diagnosis.

ELISA testing is increasingly available at major medical centers and this can detect one of the pathological antibodies (BP antigen-1) in more than 90% of patients with BP.

SPECIAL POINTS

Because a biopsy from the center of a lesion of BP rarely provides any useful diagnostic information by light microscopy, and may in fact yield false-positive results by immunofluorescence, many experts advocate the deep-shave (saucerization) excision of a small bullae intact for histological examination. A small perilesional punch may then be performed for immunofluorescence studies.

Unlike in pemphigus, it does not appear that the titers as measured by ELISA correspond to disease activity in BP.

Since BP is an antibody-mediated autoimmune condition, immunosuppressive therapies are often helpful. Prednisone is the mainstay of initial treatment, but the condition may recur when it is tapered.

Since prednisone causes significant side effects when used long term, increasingly, dermatologists use less-noxious anti-inflammatory regimens, such as combination therapy with tetracyclines and nicotinamide, as steroid-sparing agents in the management BP. These are often easily tolerated even in elderly patients.

If these more gentle regimens are not successful, more aggressive immunosuppressant agents, such as mycophenolate mofetil or azathioprine may be needed. These agents have serious potential side effects and should be managed by providers experienced in their use.

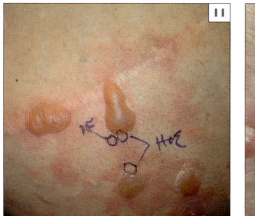

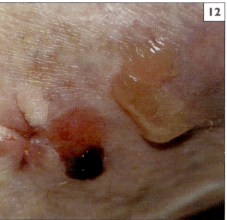

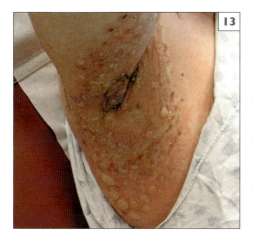

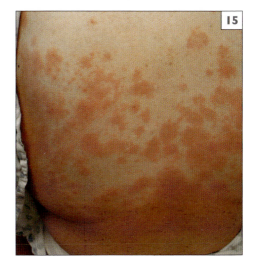

11–15 Bullous pemphigoid (**11–14**); urticarial bullous pemphigoid (**15**).

Cicatricial pemphigoid
(mucous membrane pemphigoid)

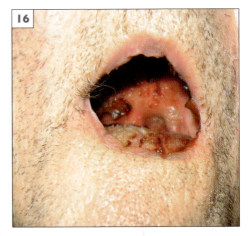

DEFINITION AND CLINICAL FEATURES
Cicatricial pemphigoid (CP), also known as mucous membrane pemphigoid, refers to a group of autoimmune blistering disorders that cause primarily erosions on mucosal services, specifically the oral mucosa and conjunctiva (**16 & 17**). The skin may also be affected, particularly that of the scalp, head and neck, the distal extremities, or the trunk (**18**).

Progressive ocular disease can lead to serious injury and symblepharon may occur. Opacification and blindness may follow long-standing, uncontrolled disease. Patients with pure ocular involvement likely constitute a distinct subset of CP patients, as do those with exclusive involvement of the scalp (Brunsting–Perry variant). Nasal involvement may present as epistaxis, crusting, and painful ulceration. Involvement of the mouth and oropharynx may include painful non-healing erosions, dysphagia, hoarseness from involvement of the vocal cords, and even esophageal stricture. The genital mucosa may be involved on occasion. It is common for CP to recur at the same sites of the body.

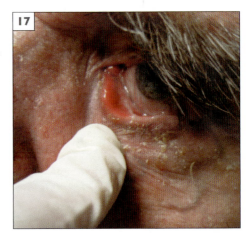

EPIDEMIOLOGY
Like bullous pemphigoid, CP is chiefly a disease of the elderly. The average age at onset is about 62–66 years. Most series have demonstrated females to be affected nearly twice as often as males. The exception to this observation involves the Brunsting–Perry variant of CP (localized only to the scalp), as these patients are nearly always elderly males. CP occurs in all races.

DIFFERENTIAL DIAGNOSIS AND INVESTIGATIONS
Other bullous skin diseases, such as pemphigus, bullous pemphigoid, bullous lupus erythematosus, epidermolysis bullosa acquisita, and porphyria cutanea tarda must be considered. Erosive oral lichen planus and even paraneoplastic pemphigus would enter the differential in cases of extreme mucosal involvement.

The diagnosis of CP is established by histological analysis. Light microscopy should be performed from the edge of a blister and direct immunofluorescence studies should be performed on perilesional skin. Light microscopy often demonstrates a dermal scar

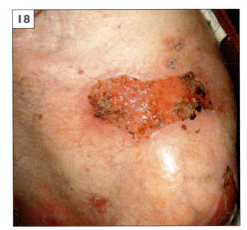

16–18 Cicatricial pemphigoid.

(hence the name 'cicatricial'), and this is not a common histological feature of bullous pemphigoid.

SPECIAL POINTS

Multidisciplinary management is necessary for patients with suspected or proven CP. Consultation with a dermatologist, ophthalmologist, and otolaryngologist is advisable. Surgical intervention by the ophthalmologist to release and reduce scarring may be needed to preserve eye function.

Treatment typically involves aggressive local and systemic immunosuppression since the scarring formed when CP is active can be disfiguring and disabling. Systemic steroids, dapsone, cyclophosphamide, mycophenolate mofetil, and azathioprine have been used with varying success. Again, these agents pose serious risks and should be used by an experienced provider.

Paraneoplastic CP has been reported in the literature. Age-appropriate cancer screening and perhaps additional testing as directed by a detailed medical history and review of systems may be beneficial for the patient.

Dermatomyositis

DEFINITION AND CLINICAL FEATURES

Classic dermatomyositis (DM) is an autoimmune connective tissue disease that may affect multiple organ systems. In the skin, DM presents with an erythematous and violaceous, photodistributed eruption of the periocular area ('heliotrope rash'), of the neck and upper chest ('shawl sign') (**19**), of the knuckle pads (Gottron's papules) (**20 & 21**) and the tendons of the forearms and elbow area (Gottron's sign) (**22**). There may also be violaceous hues to the skin of the lateral hips ('holster sign'). Pruritus, particularly of the scalp, is a common complaint. The nail folds often manifest with dilated capillaries and ragged cuticles. Cutaneous calcinosis may occur in late-stage disease in adults, and is more common in childhood cases.

Systemic involvement of DM includes marked weakness of the proximal skeletal muscles, involvement of smooth muscle with dysphagia and dysphonia, impaired intestinal motility, pulmonary fibrosis, myocarditis, and retinitis. Often patients first notice this weakness when climbing stairs, rising from a

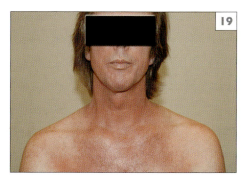

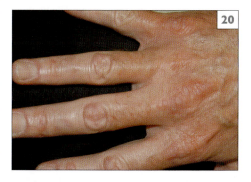

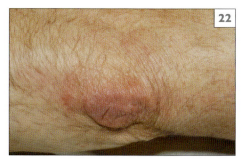

19–21 Dermatomyositis.

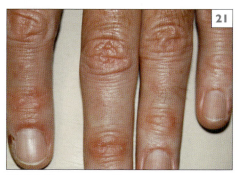

22 Dermatomyositis.

seated position, combing their hair, or reaching for items in a cabinet above shoulder level.

EPIDEMIOLOGY

DM occurs in all age groups. In children, the peak incidence for DM occurs between 5 and 10 years of age, while in adults the peak incidence occurs around 50 years of age. Females are affected twice as often as males by DM.

DIFFERENTIAL DIAGNOSIS AND INVESTIGATIONS

Systemic lupus erythematosus can cause a similar cutaneous eruption, along with systemic illness. Mixed connective tissue disease can present with findings that overlap with systemic lupus, scleroderma, and DM.

Classic DM is associated with abnormal elevations of muscle enzymes on serological testing. CK is the most sensitive enzyme for testing purposes, but AST and LDH may also be elevated. Sometimes elevated muscle enzymes precede clinical evidence of myositis. In this situation, MRI may be useful for detection of subclinical muscle inflammation. Most patients with DM have positive ANS. Antibodies of particular utility include:

- Anti-Mi-2 antibodies – highly specific for DM but insensitive as only 25% of the patients with DM demonstrate them.
- Anti-Jo-1 antibodies – more often present in patients with polymyositis than with DM, but when present they are associated with pulmonary involvement.

Skin biopsy may demonstrate an interface process and deposition of cutaneous mucin, not dissimilar from certain manifestations of cutaneous lupus. The histological findings of Gottron's papules (overlying the joints of the digits) may be particularly subtle and require expert interpretation and clinicopathological correlation.

The term 'amyopathic DM' is reserved for patients who present with the cutaneous manifestations of classic DM, but who are without clinical or laboratory evidence of muscle involvement for 2 years (although a 'provisional' diagnosis of amyopathic DM may be granted after 6 months).

SPECIAL POINTS

DM in adults, particularly those older than 60 years, can be a paraneoplastic phenomenon.

The cancers associated with DM have varied according to general prevalence of cancer in the geographic area. For example, in Asia it has often been associated with nasopharyngeal carcinoma, while in Western society it is more often associated with breast and ovarian cancer. Age-appropriate cancer screening and perhaps additional testing as directed by a detailed medical history and review of systems may be beneficial for the patient.

Treatment of DM is often a team approach involving the primary provider (who is treating the patient's general health and also performing cancer screenings), dermatologist, and rheumatologist. Topical treatment is usually not sufficient. Systemic steroids are sometimes (but not always) helpful but are difficult to use long term owing to side effects. Hydroxychloroquine and methotrexate are two commonly helpful agents. Mycophenolate mofetil, azathioprine, or other systemic immunosuppressive agents may also be helpful. These agents possess significant risks and should be prescribed by a provider experienced in treating connective tissue disease.

Acute cutaneous lupus erythematosus (systemic lupus erythematosus)

DEFINITION AND CLINICAL FEATURES

Systemic lupus erythematosus (SLE), a multisystem, autoimmune, connective tissue disease, is usually the domain of rheumatologists. However, acute presentations of lupus may be first detected within the skin. Classically the acute eruption of SLE may present as a photosensitive 'butterfly rash,' consisting of erythema across the malar cheeks and nose (**23 & 24**). Unlike seborrheic dermatitis, it does not involve the photoprotected nasolabial folds, and instead spares them. Other cutaneous manifestations may include oral or nasal ulcerations, periungual telangiectases (similar to dermatomyositis), and diffuse and non-specific alopecia.

EPIDEMIOLOGY

In the United States, the annual incidence of SLE is around 25 per 100,000 persons in the population. There is a remarkably higher prevalence of the disease in females, with multiple series demonstrating a female:male ratio of 8–15:1. SLE is particularly more common in black females and Asian females as well.

DIFFERENTIAL DIAGNOSIS AND INVESTIGATIONS

The differential diagnosis includes dermatomyositis, mixed connective tissue disease, and scleroderma.

The diagnosis of SLE is based first on the presence of serological evidence of ANS. Drug-induced cases often manifest an antihistone or anticentromere pattern. Criteria exist for use in clinical trials and include, in brief:

- Serositis/pleuritis
- Oral or nasopharyngeal ulcers
- Non-erosive arthritis
- Photosensitivity
- Anemia/leukopenia/thrombocytopenia/hypocomplementemia
- Renal compromise/dysfunction
- ANA positivity (sensitivity 99%)
- Neurological disorders/seizures/psychosis
- Skin rash (sensitivity 18%).

Skin biopsy may manifest a lichenoid infiltrate with vacuolar alterations of the basal layer of keratinocytes, and dermal mucin accumulation. A 'lupus band' along the dermoepidermal junction by direct immunofluorescence has largely been replaced by ANA/ENA serologies.

Other studies that should be considered by the primary provider or by consulting specialists include a CBC, ESR, basic metabolic panel, liver function studies, renal function studies, antiphospholipid antibodies, and coagulation function screening.

SPECIAL POINTS

Patients with acute presentations of SLE can have associated infections, thrombotic events, and neuropsychiatric complications. A high degree of suspicion is necessary for early diagnosis of these events to facilitate prompt management and to avoid complications.

Typically a patient with SLE will be primarily managed by their primary care doctor and rheumatologist. A dermatologist may be helpful in preventing and managing acute flares of skin disease, which are often associated with UV exposure. Consistent use of a wide-brimmed hat and sunscreen is critical for patients with lupus, even in the winter or on cloudy days. Special UV blocking tint for automobile glass may also be

helpful if the patient's occupation requires extensive driving.

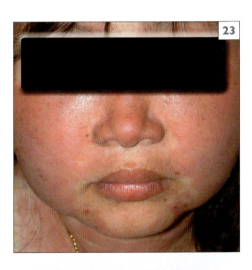

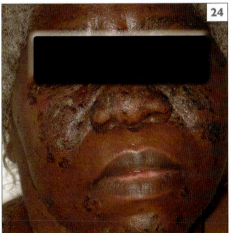

23, 24 Acute malar lupus.

Subacute cutaneous lupus erythematosus

DEFINITION AND CLINICAL FEATURES

Subacute cutaneous lupus erythematosus (SCLE) is a form of cutaneous lupus erythematosus. SCLE may occur in patients with systemic lupus erythematosus or Sjögren syndrome, and it may also be drug induced. Classically, SCLE presents in two forms: annular and psoriasiform. Both forms tend to present on the sun-exposed skin of the face, arms, and upper chest and back (in an inverted triangular pattern) (25–27). The annular form presents with erythematous rings of scaling and central clearing, somewhat akin to 'ringworm.' The psoriasiform variant presents with more uniformly erythematous and scaling plaques, similar to psoriasis, but not overlying only extensor surfaces.

EPIDEMIOLOGY

SCLE generally occurs in patients from 15 to 70 years of age with a mean age of approximately 43 years. There is a higher prevalence of the disease in females, with multiple series demonstrating a female:male ratio of 4:1. SCLE is particularly more common in white people (85%). As many as one-third of patients with SCLE may meet diagnostic criteria for systemic lupus erythematosus, although these patients may not have as fulminant and destructive end-organ damage.

DIFFERENTIAL DIAGNOSIS AND INVESTIGATIONS

The differential diagnosis includes dermatomyositis, acute systemic lupus erythematosus, and generalized discoid lupus erythematosus, as well as tinea and psoriasis (for the reasons outlined above).

The diagnosis of SCLE is based first on the presence of serological evidence of ANS. More than 80% of patients with the psoriasiform presentation of SCLE, and more than 90% of those with the annular form of SCLE, will manifest anti-Ro (SSA) autoantibodies.

Skin biopsy may manifest a lichenoid infiltrate with vacuolar alterations of the basal layer of keratinocytes, and dermal mucin accumulation. Direct immunofluorescence examination of lesional skin often demonstrates a speckled, 'dust-like' pattern within the epidermis.

Other studies that should be considered by the primary provider or by consulting specialists include a CBC, ESR, basic metabolic panel, liver function studies, and renal function studies.

SPECIAL POINTS

Treatment of SCLE is aimed at controlling symptoms and monitoring for evidence of systemic lupus. Systemic steroids are often used in short- to intermediate-length courses for flares. Vigorous sun protection with a brimmed hat and sunscreen, even on cloudy days, is required. If SCLE persists, more aggressive agents including hydroxychloroquine, mycophenolate mofetil, and azathioprine may be helpful. The risks of these agents must be weighed against the severity of the disease. If there is any suggestion of systemic lupus, a rheumatologist should be consulted.

Children of mothers with SCLE are prone to neonatal lupus and are at particular risk for congenital heart block. It is important for a female patient with SCLE to consult with her obstetrician for pre-pregnancy counseling and regularly during pregnancy.

Terbinafine, a medication that is used extensively for fungal infections including toenail infections (onychomycosis), has been associated with SCLE-like drug-induced eruptions.

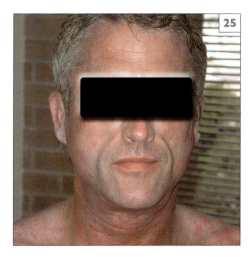

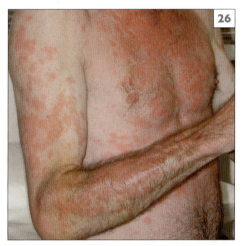

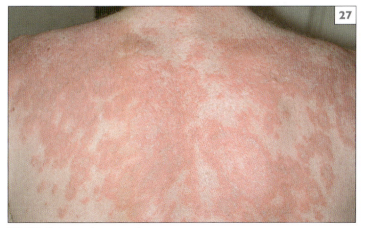

25–27 Subacute lupus erythematosus.

Discoid lupus erythematosus

DEFINITION AND CLINICAL FEATURES

Discoid lupus erythematosus (DLE) is a form of chronic cutaneous lupus erythematosus. DLE tends to involve the photoexposed areas of the head, neck and upper trunk (**28 & 29**). When it occurs beyond this area it is termed generalized DLE, and has a higher risk of systemic involvement. Classically, DLE creates indurated, erythematous, and scaling plaques that are associated with follicular plugging and central hypopigmentation with peripheral hyperpigmentation (**30**). The disease often first becomes apparent in the conchal bowls of the ear (**31**). A scarring alopecia may result. The vermillion border and even the oral mucosa may be involved as well (**32**).

EPIDEMIOLOGY

DLE typically involves a slightly younger age group than do other forms of cutaneous lupus, but it may appear in any age group. There is a higher prevalence of the disease in females, with a female:male ratio of 2:1. DLE is particularly more common in black people. Only about 5–15% of patients with DLE demonstrate any systemic involvement with their disease.

DIFFERENTIAL DIAGNOSIS AND INVESTIGATIONS

The differential diagnosis includes granuloma faciale, lichen planus, lupus vulgaris (tuberculosis), sarcoidosis, squamous cell carcinoma, and other forms of scarring alopecia.

The diagnosis of DLE is based first on a histological examination of the affected tissue. Skin biopsy may manifest vacuolar alterations of the basal layer of keratinocytes, dermal mucin accumulation, and a superficial, deep, and periadnexal inflammatory infiltrate. Overlying hyperkeratosis and follicular plugging are prominent.

Other studies that should be considered by the primary provider or by consulting specialists include a CBC, ESR, basic metabolic panel, liver function studies, and renal function studies.

SPECIAL POINTS

Given the photodistributed nature of the process, it is not very unusual for plaques of DLE to be mistaken for squamous cell carcinoma. This is particularly true when the disease presents in the elderly. On occasion, medicolegal liability has resulted when a large and disfiguring surgical procedure was performed prior to discovery of this inflammatory skin disorder, which is best managed medically.

Even small amounts of UV exposure can flare or significantly worsen DLE and for this reason patients with this disease must take great measures to avoid unnecessary exposure to the sun. Long-sleeved clothes, shirts that button high on the chest, broad-brimmed hats, and broad-spectrum (UVA and UVB blocking) sunscreens should be used. Patients should also remember that UVA passes through most standard glass and specialized window tinting is available to block it.

Since DLE is not usually associated with systemic lupus, treatment is primarily aimed at preventing and controlling symptoms. An initial workup for signs of systemic lupus is warranted for a patient with newly diagnosed DLE. High-potency topical and injected intralesional steroids are a mainstay of treatment. Typically the treatment should focus on active areas of DLE evidenced by a red or purple border. White, scar-like lesions are usually 'burned out' and do not benefit from treatment. Since DLE is a scarring process, it can cause permanent hair loss and disfigurement, so it is important to treat newly active lesions immediately. Short-course systemic steroids may be useful for widespread flares.

For more persistent or widespread disease, hydroxychloroquine is often helpful. Quinacrine, another older antimalarial, can be added to hydroxychloroquine as well. Both of these agents require regular monitoring or liver function tests and eye exams.

Thalidomide has been used in cases where other treatments have failed. It is often effective at controlling DLE but can cause numerous serious side effects and should be monitored closely by a practitioner familiar with its use. It can cause severe birth defects (including micronized or absent limbs), blood clots, neuropathy, and drowsiness. The latter three can all be accentuated in the elderly patient. Patients of child-bearing potential who are considering thalidomide treatment must be counseled on these severe risks and to use two forms of highly active birth control along with having regular pregnancy tests. Although pregnancy is unlikely in the elderly patient, it is important to remember that females in their fifties and even sixties can become pregnant.

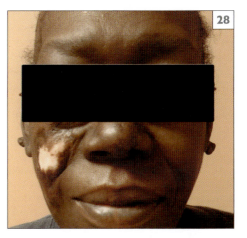

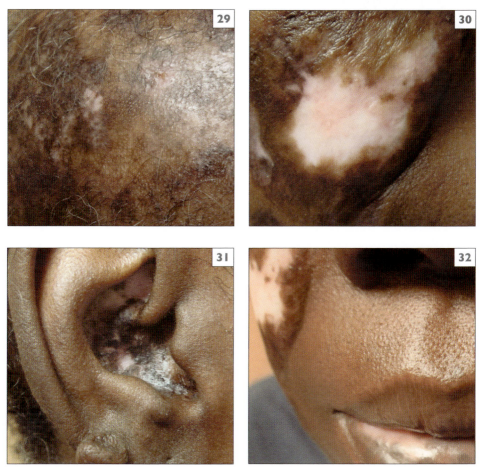

28–32 Discoid lupus erythematosus.

Scleroderma

DEFINITION AND CLINICAL FEATURES

Systemic scleroderma, a disease with visceral complications, must be distinguished from localized scleroderma, a cutaneously limited disease, better known as morphea. Morphea is chiefly a disease of childhood and early adulthood, and will not be discussed further.

Systemic scleroderma comes in two main forms: diffuse scleroderma and limited scleroderma. Diffuse scleroderma manifests not only with changes of the distal extremities and possibly the face, but also involves the proximal aspects of the extremities and the trunk. Limited scleroderma involves only areas distal to the elbow and knee, but it may involve the face and neck. In the past, most cases of limited scleroderma were called CREST syndrome (calcinosis, Raynaud phenomenon, esophageal dysmotility, sclerodactyly, and telangiectases).

Both subtypes of systemic scleroderma usually begin in the skin of the distal extremities as sclerodactyly (**33–35**), or tightness of the skin of the fingers and dorsal hands due to dermal fibrosis and sclerosis. Raynaud phenomenon of the extremities, with the characteristic and sequential white, blue, and red changes, may precede the cutaneous or systemic aspects of the disease by months or even years. Digital infarction and dry gangrene may occur due to severe vasospasm. Dilated telangiectatic capillaries of the proximal nail fold, similar to those of dermatomyositis, may be identified on close inspection (**36**). The face often demonstrates a decreased oral aperture with tightness and perioral rhytids and a 'beak-like' nose. Telangiectases may appear on the face and other areas of the skin (**37 & 38**). The skin of other affected areas typically feels tight and indurated due to fibrosis and sclerosis. Dyspigmentation of skin, often in a 'salt-and-pepper' pattern, may occur (**39**). Calcification may occur in the skin as well.

Systemic findings of scleroderma may include generalized hypertension, pulmonary hypertension, renal failure and acute hypertensive renal crisis, renal failure, congestive heart failure, pulmonary fibrosis, and esophageal dysmotility.

EPIDEMIOLOGY

Systemic sclerosis affects individuals of all races, but the risk may be slightly greater in black people, particularly young black females. In fact, the risk of systemic sclerosis is three to nine times higher in females than in males. While it may appear at any age, the peak onset occurs in individuals aged 30–50 years.

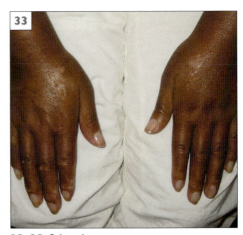

33–39 Scleroderma.

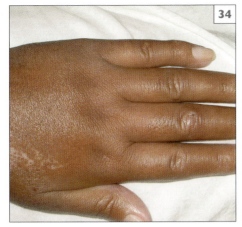

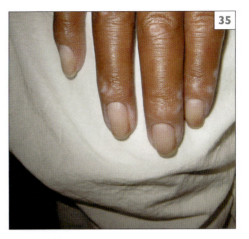

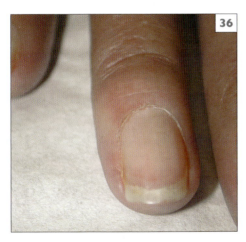

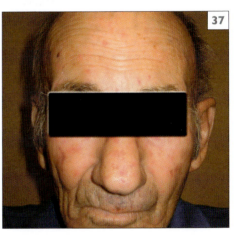

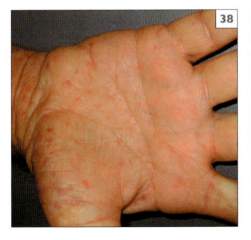

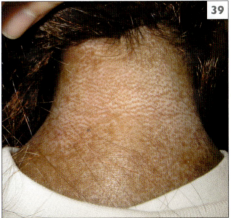

DIFFERENTIAL DIAGNOSIS AND INVESTIGATIONS

The differential diagnosis includes nephrogenic systemic fibrosis, eosinophilia–myalgia syndrome, eosinophilic fasciitis, scleromyxedema, and generalized morphea.

A skin biopsy from either subtype of systemic scleroderma (diffuse or limited), or even morphea, will show essentially identical histological features of an attenuated epidermis, dense dermal sclerosis, and entrapped adnexal structures. Clinicopathological correlation is required to ascertain the true nature and extent of the disease.

ANAs are present in about 95% of patients with systemic scleroderma. Anti-topoisomerase I antibodies (formerly anti-Scl-70) are present in approximately 30% of patients with diffuse scleroderma, but are generally absent in patients with limited scleroderma. This antibody is also associated with pulmonary fibrosis. Conversely, anti-centromere antibodies are present in about 60–90% of patients with limited scleroderma, but are rare in patients with diffuse scleroderma.

SPECIAL POINTS

Rare cases of scleroderma have been associated with occupational exposure to vinyl chloride.

Systemic scleroderma, with its protean systemic manifestations, often requires consultation with several specialists and the cooperative management of rheumatology, dermatology, pulmonology, and nephrology. Functional treatments, such as physical therapy and oxygen, may be helpful in maintaining function. Systemic treatments such as steroids, methotrexate, and immunosuppressants are usually managed by the rheumatologist and, unfortunately, often do not arrest the course of the systemic sclerosis.

Pemphigus

DEFINITION AND CLINICAL FEATURES

The term 'pemphigus' refers to a family of autoimmune blistering disorders that can affect the skin and the mucosa. Prior to the advent of exogenous corticosteroids, pemphigus had a high rate of mortality. The various types of pemphigus are as follows:

- Pemphigus vulgaris – the more common subtype, typically begins in the mouth with fragile, easily ruptured bullae which cause pain that limits oral intake (**40**). This oral involvement usually begins weeks before any skin lesions may develop. Often patients first notice an inability to tolerate foods with hard, sharp edges, such as potato or tortilla chips. The skin lesions typically consist of fragile blisters that rupture to leave eroded and weeping plaques (**41**). Indeed, the bullae of pemphigus are so superficial and fragile it is often difficult to find intact lesions on exam. More often, one identifies only a thin 'collarette' of delicate scale that represents the residua of the blister roof.
- Pemphigus foliaceous – is a less common type that is distinguished *chiefly* by the lack of mucosal involvement. Widespread fragile blisters on the face, trunk, and proximal extremities rupture to leave only erosions, peripheral scale, and central crust (**42 & 43**).
- Pemphigus vegetans – is a rare subtype of pemphigus in which heaped and vegetative lesions are present, particularly in the intertriginous areas of the body such as the axilla and inguinal folds (**44 & 45**).
- Pemphigus erythematosus – is another rare subtype of pemphigus in which there are overlapping features of pemphigus and lupus erythematosus.
- Paraneoplastic pemphigus (**149**) – is a form of pemphigus particularly associated with non-Hodgkin lymphoma. By definition, paraneoplastic pemphigus has intense ulcerative and painful stomatitis as a key feature. The mortality rates for this form of the disease approaches 90%, with death often the result of sepsis, with multiorgan failure, or respiratory failure due to the direct effects of the disease on the respiratory tract epithelium.

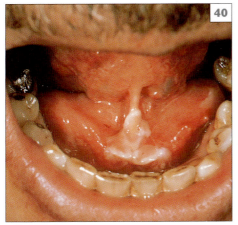

40 Oral pemphigus.

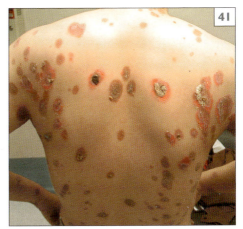

41 Pemphigus vulgaris.

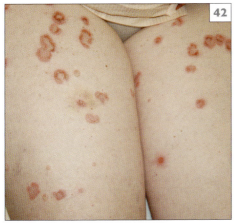

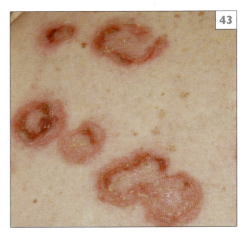

42, 43 Pemphigus foliaceous.

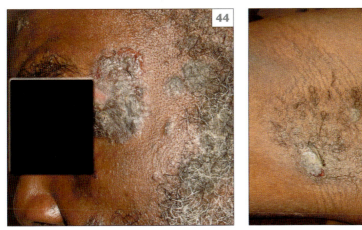

44, 45 Pemphigus vegetans.

EPIDEMIOLOGY

All races may be affected by pemphigus, although the Jewish population seems to be particularly affected. In adults, males and females are affected equally. Pemphigus may affect persons of all ages, although in general, pemphigus is not as common in elderly patients as is bullous pemphigoid. For most forms of pemphigus the average age of onset is between the fifth and sixth decades of life. Paraneoplastic pemphigus is more common in the elderly, where the mean age at onset is 60 years.

DIFFERENTIAL DIAGNOSIS AND INVESTIGATIONS

The differential diagnosis includes bullous pemphigoid, erosive oral lichen planus, extensive bullous impetigo, and seborrheic dermatitis (for pemphigus foliaceous on the face).

Skin biopsy in pemphigus vulgaris and pemphigus foliaceous demonstrates intraepidermal vesiculation caused by acantholysis (discohesion of keratinocytes). Often a significant number of eosinophils are present in the blister cavity and the surrounding superficial dermis. In pemphigus vegetans, the epidermis is often acanthotic (thickened) and eosinophilic crypts are present in the epidermis.

Direct immunofluorescence examination of perilesional skin demonstrates the 'net-like' deposition of immunoreactants within the epidermis. In pemphigus erythematosus, direct immunofluorescence often demonstrates the net-like deposition of pemphigus and a band-like pattern of deposition along the dermoepidermal junction that is consistent with lupus erythematosus.

ELISA testing, where available, demonstrates circulating antibodies in about 90% of persons with the classic forms of pemphigus, and, unlike bullous pemphigoid, the titers often correspond to disease activity.

In contrast to the other forms of pemphigus, paraneoplastic disease usually demonstrates a lichenoid inflammatory infiltrate with interface reaction and the direct killing of keratinocytes by lymphocytes along the dermoepidermal junction. Also, unlike other forms of pemphigus, indirect immunofluorescence examination of the patient's serum using rat bladder as a substrate is typically positive, and often this is used as a screening examination.

SPECIAL POINTS

Prior to the invention of systemic steroids, systemic pemphigus was usually a fatal condition. Treatment is important to suppress blister formation and maintain function of the aerodigestive tract.

Initial treatment of all forms of pemphigus usually involves systemic steroids, often in high doses. Patients with more severe forms may need long-term, low-dose steroids even while also using steroid-sparing agents. In cases of long-term steroid use, monitoring for potential side effects (including infections, bone loss, fractures, diabetes, weight gain, fluid retention, hypertension, and stomach ulcers) should be pursued regularly. Concomitant use of oral calcium, vitamin D supplementation, and regular weight-bearing exercise is often recommended. Oral bisphosphonate medications may also slow bone loss.

Commonly used steroid-sparing agents include dapsone, mycophenolate mofetil, and azathioprine. More severe or recalcitrant cases may benefit from IVIG or rituximab, both of which may decrease the levels of circulating antibodies that cause the disease.

Fogo sevalgem is a form of endemic pemphigus foliaceous occurring in the Amazon basin of South America. It is thought to be related to an infectious vector or other substance leading to molecular mimicry that is related to the bite of the black fly in the jungles of this area. Other than this geographic confinement, fogo sevalgem appears, clinically and histologically, identical to pemphigus foliaceous.

Sjögren syndrome

DEFINITION AND CLINICAL FEATURES

Sjögren syndrome, also known as sicca complex, is a chronic autoimmune disorder characterized by xerostomia (dry mouth), xerophthalmia (dry eyes) (**46**), and lymphocytic infiltration of the exocrine glands. Additional cutaneous manifestations of Sjögren syndrome include:

- Dryness and scaling of the skin
- Partial or complete anhidrosis
- Dry, sparse, and brittle hair leading to diffuse alopecia
- Erythema of the nose and cheeks may be present
- Annular erythematous and scaling rash on the face and neck
- Sjögren vasculitis (a form of leukocytoclastic vasculitis), typically on the lower legs (formerly Waldenström purpura) (**221–223**).

Additionally, patients with Sjögren syndrome have overlapping and/or associated acute systemic lupus erythematosus, subacute cutaneous lupus erythematosus, scleroderma or mixed connective tissue disease, and rheumatoid arthritis.

EPIDEMIOLOGY

Sjögren syndrome occurs in all races. Females are affected much more often than are males, with a female:male ratio of 9:1. While the disease may occur at any age, it most often first presents in persons aged 30–50 years. Sjögren syndrome is exquisitely rare if ever present in children.

DIFFERENTIAL DIAGNOSIS AND INVESTIGATIONS

Rosacea can cause dry and itchy eyes. Cicatricial pemphigoid, while ultimately causing mucosal ulceration, can begin as a dry sensation in the eyes. The overlap of Sjögren syndrome with systemic lupus erythematosus, subacute cutaneous lupus erythematosus, and scleroderma means that all these diseases lie in the differential diagnosis as well.

No single test is sufficient, sensitive, or specific to diagnose Sjögren syndrome, and clinicopathological correlation is always needed. Measurements by the ophthalmologist or oral specialist to quantify lacrimal (Schirmer test) or salivary gland output may be a first step in suggesting the diagnosis.

An excisional biopsy from the inside of the lower lip may demonstrate focal lymphocytic sialadenitis, defined as dense aggregates of >50 lymphocytes in perivascular and/or periductal locations. This may be graded by an experienced histopathologist so as to give a strong indication as to the likelihood of Sjögren syndrome. Nevertheless, because of the large size of the sample required, it should not be undertaken lightly, and should be performed only where the pre-test clinical probability is high.

SPECIAL POINTS

In dermatology, the particular relevance of Sjögren syndrome lies in the overlap and association that the disease has with systemic lupus erythematosus, subacute cutaneous lupus erythematosus, scleroderma, and in connective tissue disease-associated leukocytoclastic vasculitis. A thorough history and workup for these conditions, along with consultation with a rheumatologist, are often helpful in a newly diagnosed patient.

Treatment depends on the severity of the disease. Artificial tear and saliva products are available to help with chronic dryness. The skin will often require repeated use of thick moisturizers, such as petrolatum.

Patients with Sjögren syndrome have an increased incidence of B-cell non-Hodgkin lymphoma.

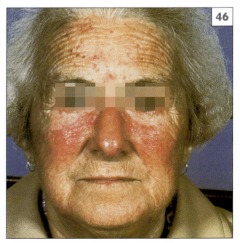

46 Dry eyes of Sjögren syndrome. From Lewis & Jordan: *A Colour Handbook of Oral Medicine*, Manson Publishing, 2004.

NEUTROPHILIC DERMATOSES

Sweet syndrome

DEFINITION AND CLINICAL FEATURES

Sweet syndrome, also known as acute febrile neutrophilic dermatosis, is a reaction pattern that occurs in response to a variety of systemic factors, including hematological disease, infection, inflammation, connective tissue disease, or drug/vaccination exposure.

Typically a moderate fever precedes the cutaneous eruption by several days. Skin lesions consist of erythematous to violaceous papules, plaques, or nodules. The lesions are often located on the face, neck, and extremities (**47 & 48**). Dermal edema can be substantial, leading to a mammillated plaque or producing a pseudovesicular appearance. Sweet syndrome demonstrates pathergy, where lesions occur in areas of minor trauma, including venepuncture. On the other hand, there is substantial overlap between bullous Sweet syndrome and pyoderma gangrenosum, another neutrophilic dermatosis, and some experts consider them to be essentially a single pathological process (neutrophilic dermatosis of the dorsal hands). Headaches, malaise, and arthralgias are also common.

Sweet syndrome is associated with a malignancy, particularly a hemopoietic disorder like acute myeloid leukemia, in up to 20–25% of cases. Presence of anemia or thrombocytopenia during an episode increases the likelihood of an associated hemopoietic malignancy. Associated inflammatory diseases, such as inflammatory bowel disease, lupus erythematosus, and rheumatoid arthritis, can be identified in about 15% of patients. Use of granulocyte–monocyte colony-stimulating factor, as well as other medications, may also promote an eruption.

Patients with Sweet syndrome often have multiple or repeated episodes related to a common trigger.

EPIDEMIOLOGY

Sweet syndrome occurs in patients of all races. Classic Sweet syndrome is more common in females, with a female:male ratio of 2–3:1, but in malignancy-associated disease this female predilection is lost. Classic Sweet syndrome occurs most often in patients 30–50 years of age, but again in malignancy-associated disease it may be more common in older individuals.

DIFFERENTIAL DIAGNOSIS AND INVESTIGATIONS

The differential diagnosis of Sweet syndrome includes other neutrophilic dermatoses, particularly pyoderma gangrenosum when there are bullous lesions on the feet, granuloma annulare, erythema multiforme, erythema nodosum, and Behçet disease.

Diagnostic criteria have been proposed and include two major and two minor criteria, the major criteria being:

- Abrupt onset of erythema and tender or painful plaques or nodules (occasionally with vesicles, pustules, or bullae)
- Dermal neutrophilic infiltration without leukocytoclastic vasculitis.

The minor criteria are:

- Preceding non-specific respiratory or gastrointestinal infection, associated inflammatory disease, hemopoietic disorder, solid tumor, pregnancy, or medication exposure/vaccination
- Episodic malaise and fever (>38°C)
- Three of four laboratory findings including elevated ESR (>20 mm), C-reactive protein, elevated peripheral neutrophils, or leukocytosis
- Excellent response to systemic corticosteroids or potassium iodide.

Practically speaking, a skin biopsy should be performed to confirm the diagnosis, and often the diagnosis is first suggested by the dermatopathologist. Histopathological findings include a dense superficial neutrophilic infiltrate with papillary dermal edema. True vasculitis is not identified.

Bone marrow aspiration should be considered if the patient is elderly, particularly if the CBC is abnormally low. It should also be considered in all cases of atypical bullous or ulcerative Sweet syndrome. Age-appropriate cancer screening and evaluation for inflammatory bowel disease are indicated if no other underlying cause is found, again particularly if the patient presents with atypical bullous or ulcerative lesions.

SPECIAL POINTS

Treatment of Sweet syndrome is aimed at resolving and preventing the nodules. It is critical to exclude an underlying leukemia or myelodysplastic syndrome when a patient has a neutrophilic dermatosis.

Systemic steroids are often quickly helpful in improving a flare, but a poor choice for long-term maintenance due to side effects. Medications that control neutrophils such as dapsone and colchicine are often used as steroid-sparing agents.

47, 48 Sweet syndrome.

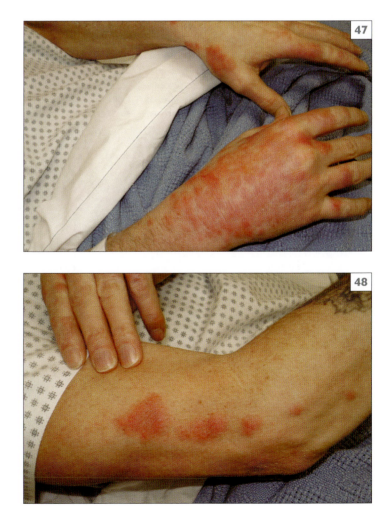

Pyoderma gangrenosum

DEFINITION AND CLINICAL FEATURES

Pyoderma gangrenosum (PG) is an unusual neutrophilic dermatosis of unclear etiology which leads to sterile ulcerations that heal slowly with significant scarring. Typically PG begins as a small, red papule or pustule that evolves, often relentlessly, into a larger ulcerative lesion (**49 & 50**). Pain can be intense and is often a key historical feature. Arthralgias and malaise may also be present. Commonly patients insist that they have been bitten by a brown recluse or other spider, but offer no other evidence of such an event.

Systemic illness exists in about 50% of patients with PG. Associated diseases include inflammatory bowel disease, leukemia or other hemopoietic disorders, rheumatoid arthritis, and other connective tissue diseases including lupus erythematosus and Sjögren syndrome.

The ulcerations of PG are often deep and undermined, with prominent surrounding violaceous erythema. The leg is a common site, as PG, like Sweet syndrome, demonstrates pathergy and may occur in areas subjected to minor (and often unrecalled) trauma. Superficial variants of PG may occur on the hands and overlap with bullous or ulcerative Sweet syndrome. Unusual perioral forms (pyostomatitis vegetans) and genital forms of PG exist as well.

EPIDEMIOLOGY

PG occurs in all races, and both sexes. A slight female predominance is debated. While PG may occur at any age, it commonly first presents in the fourth and fifth decades.

DIFFERENTIAL DIAGNOSIS AND INVESTIGATIONS

The differential diagnosis includes ecthyma, ecthyma gangrenosum, Sweet syndrome, vasculitis, and venous or arterial ulcers.

Spider bites, particularly those of the brown recluse spider, pose a particular diagnostic challenge. Patients, often due to the lack of any other firm explanation in lay understanding, become convinced that they have been bitten, even despite lack of evidence of such an event. In this regard, knowledge of the

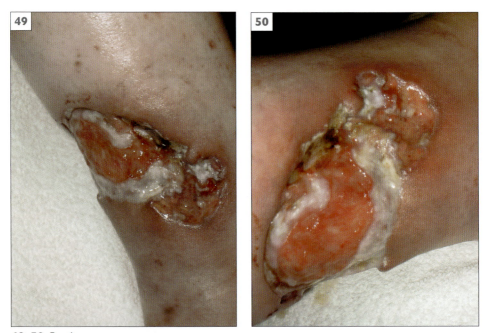

49, 50 Pyoderma gangrenosum.

local flora and fauna is useful. For example, brown recluse spiders are not present in Colorado, the home of one of the authors; a travel history would be requisite for this to be a possibility in this practice area.

There is no single diagnostic test to include PG. A tissue biopsy from the edge of the ulcer demonstrates an undermined and ragged epidermis with an underlying dense neutrophilic infiltrate within the dermis. Special stains may be performed on the tissue to exclude an infectious process. Cultures on the tissue are also advisable.

SPECIAL POINTS
It is important that consideration of PG be made for all skin ulcers, although it is usually a diagnosis of exclusion. PG demonstrates pathergy (it can develop at sites of injury such as blood draw sites or minor trauma). Debridement of the ulcer, often beneficial for ulcers of many varied etiologies, leads only to continued enlargement when the ulcer is caused by PG. There are cases where a patient was gravely harmed by continued debridement of undetected PG.

Once infectious and neoplastic causes of ulceration have been excluded, aggressive immunosuppressive treatment is usually required. Systemic steroids (such as high-dose prednisone) are best for initial treatment. Steroids will usually quickly improve the ulcers and may then be tapered. Recurrence during or after tapering can be treated with further steroids, but the long-term complications must be considered. Steroid-sparing agents commonly used in PG include dapsone, mycophenolate mofetil, and azathioprine. When these fail or cannot be tolerated, infliximab has also shown success.

ALLERGIC AND HYPERSENSITIVITY PROCESSES

Drug eruptions

DEFINITION AND CLINICAL FEATURES
A drug eruption, as a hypersensitivity process, can occur in almost any patient in response to almost any medication. Typically drug eruptions present as a symmetric, largely blanchable, erythematous macular, maculopapular, or morbilliform (resembling measles) type of eruption (**51**).

More than 95% of all drug eruptions are due to delayed-type hypersensitivity processes, with less than 5% of drug eruptions being IgE-based immediate reactions. Typically these delayed-type hypersensitivity drug eruptions begin 7–20 days after the medication is started. Peripheral hypereosinophilia is persuasive evidence for a drug eruption, when present, but its absence does not foreclose the possibility of a drug-mediated hypersensitivity process.

While generally new medications are most likely to be implicated in a drug reaction, it is important to note that drug reactions can occur even after years of use, seemingly without prior difficulty. Some commonly prescribed medications, such as TMP/SMX and ampicillin/amoxicillin may yield a drug reaction in up to 5% of patients exposed.

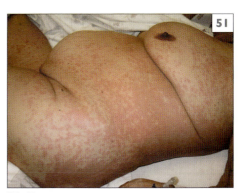

51 Drug eruption.

EPIDEMIOLOGY

Drug eruptions are more common in the elderly, particularly those already taking multiple medications (polypharmacy). Immunocompromised persons often have a higher risk of developing a drug eruption than does the general population. For example, HIV-positive patients with a CD4 count <200 cells/μL have a 10- to 50-fold increased risk of developing a drug eruption to TMP/SMX.

DIFFERENTIAL DIAGNOSIS AND INVESTIGATIONS

Simple urticaria, viral exanthems, and early presentations of more complex and dangerous drug-induced eruptions, such as Stevens–Johnson syndrome or toxic epidermal necrolysis, must be considered in the differential diagnosis.

Generally a detailed medication history, paying particular attention to medications initiated in the previous 1–3 weeks, will provide important diagnostic information.

To distinguish a simple drug eruption from a more serious drug-induced process, as outlined above, the following points of the physical exam should be reviewed by the provider and specifically evaluated and commented on:

- Mucous membrane erosions or ulcerations (conjunctival, oral, genital)
- Presence of any bullae on the body
- Presence of a Nikolsky sign (shearing of the epidermis with lateral pressure; indicates serious eruption that may constitute a medical emergency)
- Erythroderma (confluent erythema)
- Angioedema or tongue swelling
- Purpura (non-blanching eruption)
- Skin necrosis
- Lymphadenopathy
- High fever, respiratory distress, hypotension.

Skin biopsy may demonstrate a superficial perivascular lymphocytic infiltrate, possibly with eosinophils, but these findings are not exclusively diagnostic of a drug eruption, and the chief utility of such a test may be in excluding other processes.

Other important laboratory investigations to be considered include a CBC (to evaluate for eosinophilia or leukopenia), liver function studies, and a basic metabolic panel.

SPECIAL POINTS

Treatment for drug eruptions primarily consists of removing the offending drug. Doing so should involve consultation with the primary doctor and the doctor who prescribed the drug to avoid sudden discontinuation of important treatments. It is also important to check for medications in the same class or that cross-react with the offending agent to avoid recurrence.

Just as minor drug eruptions can be slow to develop, generally occurring 7–20 days after beginning a new medication, they are also slow to resolve, even after cessation of the offending agent. Because a complex immunological cascade is involved in the mechanism, it is not unusual for symptoms to continue to plateau for 2–3 days after discontinuance before improvement becomes apparent.

While waiting for improvement after the drug has been discontinued, topical or systemic steroids may be temporarily helpful. Treatments for general itching such as antihistamines (especially sedating antihistamines such as hydroxyzine or doxepin) and oatmeal baths may be helpful symptomatically.

Acute generalized exanthematous pustulosis

DEFINITION AND CLINICAL FEATURES

Acute generalized exanthematous pustulosis (AGEP) is a specific type of hypersensitivity process which consists of erythematous macules that quickly become studded with small pustules that are not follicularly based. The face and flexural/intertriginous areas of the body are chiefly affected (**52 & 53**). AGEP has been described as a reaction to numerous medications, exogenous ingestions including illicit drugs, and occasionally secondary to infections. Many cases are associated with the use of beta-lactam or macrolide antibiotics.

AGEP typically begins about 1–2 days after the initiation of the offending medication. The pustules that result resolve over 9–10 days with discontinuance of the medication. Associated symptoms may include pruritus, fever, and peripheral eosinophilia.

EPIDEMIOLOGY

AGEP can occur in all races and ages. There does not appear to be any predisposition based on sex.

DIFFERENTIAL DIAGNOSIS AND INVESTIGATIONS

The differential diagnosis would include pustular psoriasis, folliculitis (which is follicularly centered), miliaria pustulosa, subcorneal pustulosis, tinea, and other drug eruptions.

Skin biopsy of AGEP usually demonstrates spongiosis, and intraepidermal pustules and eosinophils in the underlying dermal infiltrate. The presence of eosinophils in the biopsy is useful as it makes the diagnosis of psoriasis unlikely.

Other laboratory testing useful for evaluation of any drug-based process may be considered to evaluate AGEP as well.

SPECIAL POINTS

Treatment for AGEP is solely based on identifying and removing the offending drug. Symptomatic treatments with oral or topical steroids, antihistamines, and oatmeal baths may help if itching is a problem.

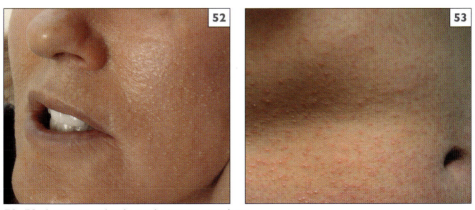

52, 53 Acute generalized exanthematous pustulosis.

Stevens–Johnson syndrome/toxic epidermal necrolysis

DEFINITION AND CLINICAL FEATURES

Stevens–Johnson syndrome (SJS) and toxic epidermal necrolysis (TEN) are serious and potentially life-threatening hypersensitivity processes, generally attributable to ingestions and, in particular, medications. In particular sulfa drugs, antiepileptics, and antibiotics are the most common causes of this combined reaction pattern. Infections may be associated with some cases, particularly with SJS.

SJS/TEN is now considered by most authorities to be spectrums of disease placed on a continuum. In brief, the most widely accepted definition of SJS/TEN is:

- SJS – requires involvement of at least two of three mucosal surfaces (conjunctival, oropharyngeal, genital) (**54 & 55**) along with erythematous and generally targetoid lesions on the trunk and extremities (**56 & 57**), but with <10% BSA involved.
- TEN – requires generally the same type of mucosal involvement, but has skin involvement of >30% BSA.
- SJS/TEN overlap – as above but with an intermediate 10–30% BSA involved.

Within 4–5 days to 3 weeks after the start of the offending drug, most patients with SJS/TEN develop first a prodrome of malaise, fever,

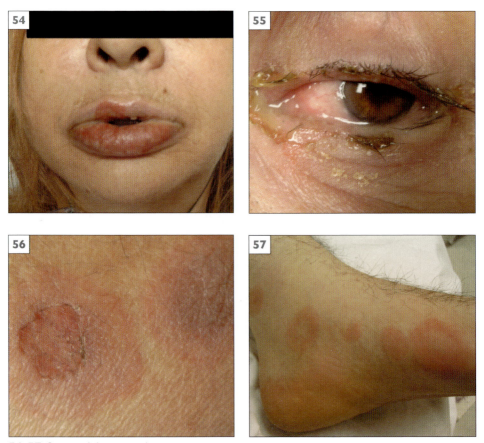

54–57 Stevens–Johnson syndrome.

headache, cough, and conjunctivitis. Targetoid erythematous macules develop and then, over 1–3 days, the epidermis is sloughed leading to large flaccid bullae. The nails and eyebrows may also be lost with the sloughed epithelium.

In TEN, large sheets of epidermis may be sloughed with minimal lateral shearing pressure (Nikolsky sign), exposing weepy, painful, and erythematous skin. Bronchial epithelium may also slough, leading to cough, dyspnea, pneumonia, and hypoxemia. Pulmonary edema, renal failure, hepatitis, and end-organ failure may develop. The significant loss of skin may lead to massive water loss and dysregulation of body temperature.

The prognosis for SJS is relatively good, with an approximately 5% mortality rate. With TEN, the prognosis is decidedly more guarded, with a mortality rate often exceeding 50% or more, depending on the percentage BSA involved and any existing comorbidities.

EPIDEMIOLOGY

Of course, the epidemiology of SJS and TEN is also clouded by differences in disease definitions. Considering SJS/TEN together, the crude incidence is probably about two cases per million people per year, but cases of SJS likely outnumber TEN by about three to one. While SJS/TEN can occur in any age group, the mean age of patients with SJS has varied from 25 to 45 years, and the mean age of patients with TEN has been reported to be between 45 and 65 years. There are no known racial predilections. For reasons that are not well understood, patients with HIV infection have been reported to have an approximately three-fold increased risk of SJS/TEN.

DIFFERENTIAL DIAGNOSIS AND INVESTIGATIONS

The differential diagnosis of SJS/TEN includes erythematous drug eruptions, phototoxic eruptions, staphylococcal scalded skin syndrome, toxic shock syndrome, and acute generalized exanthematous pustulosis.

Skin biopsy is useful in excluding or including many of these conditions, but results may be delayed in comparison to the urgency of the situation. Frozen-section examination of sloughed epidermis may be useful in distin-guishing TEN from staphylococcal scalded skin syndrome, as TEN will manifest a subepidermal split and full-thickness epidermal necrosis, while only partial-thickness epidermal sloughing and minimal keratinocyte necrosis will be noted in staphylococcal scalded skin syndrome.

SJS/TEN is a medical emergency, and if it is suspected consultation with an expert and admission to a burn unit or intensive care unit are advised. Often one of the earliest indications of SJS/TEN may be skin pain (rather than pruritus) out of proportion to that expected from a simple drug eruption. Also, the involvement of mucosal surfaces is another key feature and is the basis for careful inspection of the conjunctiva, oral mucosa, and genital mucosa every time a drug reaction is suspected. A positive Nikolsky sign, or sloughing of the skin with lateral pressure, is also useful in suggesting the strong possibility of SJS/TEN in comparison to a simple drug eruption.

SPECIAL POINTS

A prognostic scoring system (SCORTEN), based on seven independent and easily measured clinical and laboratory variables, has been developed and validated for use in SJS/TEN. Published survival curves corresponding to the SCORTEN analysis are useful to clinicians when discussing a patient's prognosis with family members or medical staff.

Patients with SJS/TEN should be immediately transferred to a facility with a burn ICU that is experienced in the care of this dangerous condition, as close attention to dressing changes, monitoring, and infection is required. Immediately stopping the offending medication is critical. Numerous treatments have been tried, including systemic steroids, IVIG, and cyclosporine, but none has shown convincing success.

PHOTORELATED CONDITIONS

Polymorphous light eruption

DEFINITION AND CLINICAL FEATURES

Polymorphous light eruption (PMLE) is the single most common photorelated dermatosis, although it is less common in elderly than in younger patients. As the name implies, the condition is polymorphous, but it typically consists of pruritic, erythematous papules coalescing into plaques on the photoexposed face, neck, upper extremities, and upper trunk (**58**). Generally, the lesions develop 30 min to several hours after UV exposure and then resolve over several days. For most patients with PMLE, the condition is worse in the early spring and improves throughout the summer and fall due to skin 'hardening.'

EPIDEMIOLOGY

It is thought that PMLE exists in about 10% of the US population, but often the condition is subclinical or, at least, it is not recognized by the patient as being related to sunlight exposure. Females appear to be three times more likely to be affected than males. Usually PMLE has its onset in the first three decades of life, but males may often have a later onset of disease. All racial types are affected by PMLE, but this condition must be distinguished from actinic prurigo (also known as PMLE of Native Americans), which is more common in persons of native North and South American heritage.

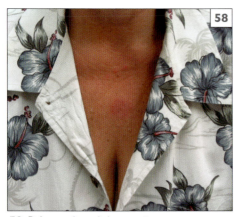

58 Polymorphous light eruption.

DIFFERENTIAL DIAGNOSIS AND INVESTIGATIONS

PMLE must be distinguished chiefly from solar urticaria (an immediate phenomenon occurring within minutes of sunlight exposure), rosacea (often worsened by the sun but unexpected on the arms), and phototoxic/photoallergic eruptions.

There is no single diagnostic test for PMLE. Classically, the skin biopsy of PMLE shows a superficial and deep perivascular lymphocytic inflammatory infiltrate with prominent papillary edema. This is in contrast to phototoxic eruptions which often demonstrate necrotic keratinocytes within the epidermis. Challenge reactions can be initiated which replicate the eruption in response to purposefully dosed UV light exposure.

SPECIAL POINTS

It is thought that females may be particularly predisposed to PMLE because certain estrogens inhibit immunosuppression that normally accompanies exposure to UV light.

Treatment is usually short-term oral steroids at times of outbreaks (such as on a sunny vacation). Vigorous sun protection may prevent outbreaks. Repeated occurrences may benefit with 'hardening' using narrow-band or PUVA phototherapy in the early spring, which will often keep a patient clear all summer.

Phototoxic/Photoallergic reactions

DEFINITION AND CLINICAL FEATURES

Phototoxic eruptions are caused by direct toxic interaction between a photoactivated chemical and the skin. The classic example of this would be lime juice, which, when placed on the skin and exposed to sunlight, forms coumarins, which are directly toxic to the skin and produce a phytophotodermatitis. This is often seen in vacationers drinking lime-based or lime-accessorized drinks poolside and unwittingly getting the juice on the skin. The result is erythematous, pruritic, and hyperpigmented eruptions assuming bizarre configurations on the skin, often in the shapes of digits or with 'drip-marks' (**59**).

Conversely, photoallergic reactions are not directly toxic to the skin. Instead, the chemical, in the presence of sunlight, forms a photoallergen that then goes on to yield effects through the activation of the immunological cascade. In this regard, it is simply a different form of allergic contact dermatitis, but UV light is necessary to yield the allergen. Because the immunological system is involved in the reaction only a small amount of the photoallergen is needed in comparison to phototoxicity. Oxybenzone, a component of some sunscreens, is the most common photoallergen.

Medications can increase one's photosensitivity by being either a phototoxin or through photoallergic mechanisms or both. Common medications leading to increased photosensitivity that are often used in the elderly are shown in *Table 1*.

EPIDEMIOLOGY
Both phototoxic and photoallergic eruptions can occur at any age and within any race. In general, phototoxic eruptions are more prevalent than photoallergic conditions.

DIFFERENTIAL DIAGNOSIS AND INVESTIGATIONS
Certainly the chief point of discrimination in phototoxic and photoallergic reactions is simply separating one from the other. In truth, it is of lesser consequence than one might think, as the correct advice for either condition is to avoid exposure.

SPECIAL POINTS
While oxybenzone, a constituent of sunscreens, is the most common photoallergen, it is actually a well-tolerated product with a low relative rate of allergenicity. Nevertheless, it is the sheer volume of use among persons with prolonged and purposeful sun exposure that makes it the most common photoallergen.

Of course, treatment of these reactions depends on removing the offending allergen. A careful history (including the patient's hobbies and occupation) can isolate potential suspects. Patch testing may be helpful in identifying allergens and photopatch testing in identifying photoallergens.

Table 1 Common medications leading to increased photosensitivity	Phototoxin	Photoallergen
Antibiotics		
Tetracyclines	Yes	No
Fluoroquinolones	Yes	No
TMP/SMX	Yes	No
NSAIDs*	Yes	Yes
Diuretics		
Furosemide	Yes	No
Hydrochlorothiazide	Yes	Yes
Cardiac medications		
Amiodarone	Yes	No
Diltiazem	Yes	No
Quinidine	Yes	Yes
Other		
Sulfonylurea	No	Yes

*Some NSAIDs are only phototoxins, others are only photoallergens, and others are both, yet nearly all NSAIDs are photosensitizers.

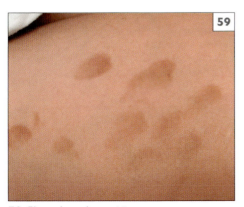

59

59 Phytophotodermatitis.

Chronic actinic dermatitis
(actinic reticuloid)

DEFINITION AND CLINICAL FEATURES

Chronic actinic dermatitis (CAD) is a unifying term used to describe a persistent and eczematous eruption involving principally sun-exposed skin. The three main criteria of CAD are:

- Reduced phototolerance (often as measured by the minimal dose of UVA to induce erythema)
- Persistent eczematous eruption that predominantly affects sun-exposed skin and sometimes extends to covered areas
- Histopathological changes consistent with chronic eczema often with changes resembling cutaneous lymphoma.

CAD usually begins as persistent erythema of the face (**60 & 61**), with later development of eczematous and heavily lichenified eruption on all sun-exposed skin, including the hands (**62 & 63**). With time, even non-sun-exposed areas may be involved. Intense pruritus, with resultant scratching, may lead to alopecia, including loss of the eyebrows. This heavy manipulation of the skin may lead to such profound changes of lichenification that a leonine facies results.

EPIDEMIOLOGY

CAD is most common in temperate climates, but it may occur in people of all races. The condition is classically seen in elderly males and is rare in females.

DIFFERENTIAL DIAGNOSIS AND INVESTIGATIONS

The differential diagnosis might include other forms of dermatitis, drug photosensitivity, polymorphic light eruption, or even leprosy (given the leonine facies).

Skin biopsy demonstrates spongiosis, acanthosis, and a dense mononuclear-cell infiltrate. Not infrequently, this mononuclear infiltrate manifests large, hyperchromatic, and convoluted nuclei. In this respect, CAD may be difficult to differentiate from cutaneous T-cell lymphoma; however, CAD characteristically has a predominance of CD8 cells in the epidermis, while cutaneous lymphoma is nearly always, not invariably, a CD4-based process. Phototesting using UV and even visible radiation demonstrates hypersensitivity and a reduced MED.

Patch testing to other compounds may be of utility, as allergic and/or photoallergic contact dermatitis often coexists and may predate the changes of CAD. Sensitivity to sesquiterpene lactone (presence in Compositae plants), fragrance compounds, colophony, and rubber accelerators is common in patients with CAD. This pre-existing photoallergic disposition may be involved in the development of CAD, which is otherwise poorly understood. Avoidance of photoallergens may prevent significant worsening.

SPECIAL POINTS

One theory regarding development of CAD has proposed that during an initial photoallergic reaction, a normal skin constituent is altered to become antigenic. Accordingly, as the disease progresses, UV radiation alone, without the photoallergen, may trigger the immune response and propagate the disease.

Treatment of CAD can be challenging. Vigorous sun protection with a brimmed hat and sunscreen is critical, even on cloudy days. Systemic steroids may help with short-term flairs but are not a good long-term choice. Systemic immunosuppressives such as cyclosporine and mycophenolate mofetil can be helpful. Given that many of these patients have a long history of sun exposure, long-term immunosuppression may significantly increase the risk of skin cancer.

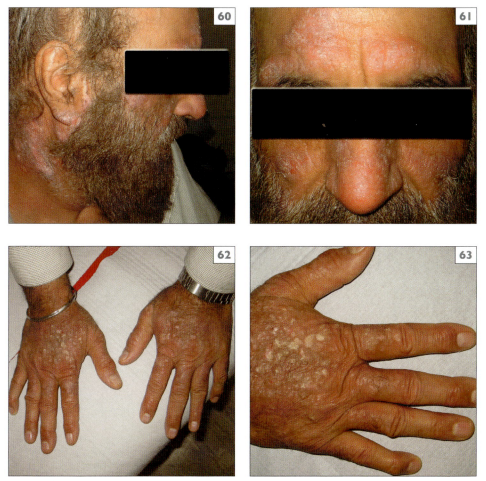

60– 63 Chronic actinic dermatitis.

Porphyria cutanea tarda

DEFINITION AND CLINICAL FEATURES

Porphyria cutanea tarda (PCT) is the most common form of porphyria. In the acquired subtype individuals with a genetic predisposition to develop PCT do so after exposure to conditions that promote iron overload (alcoholism, oral contraceptives), after exposure to hepatotoxins, or in the context of hepatic tumors (hepatoma). Decreased hepatic expression of uroporphyrinogen decarboxylase, an important enzyme in the heme synthesis pathway, leads to an accumulation of toxic porphyrins, yielding the disease.

Cutaneous manifestations of PCT include thin and fragile skin of the photoexposed face and hands (**64**). Bullae form in these areas and the resultant scarring leads ultimately to milia formation (**65**). There is often hypertrichosis of the periocular areas of the face (**66**). Uroporphyrins may lead to sclerodermoid changes of the skin in about 20% of patients with PCT.

Pseudoporphyria is a condition caused by some medications, which produces the clinical and histological findings of porphyria. Only laboratory testing can distinguish porphyria from pseudoporphyria.

EPIDEMIOLOGY

PCT occurs in persons of all races. PCT typically develops in middle to late adulthood. Prior to the advent of oral contraceptives, iron deficiency secondary to heavy menses made PCT less common in females. Other conditions of iron overload, such as alcoholism and hemochromatosis, predispose to the unmasking of PCT in susceptible individuals.

DIFFERENTIAL DIAGNOSIS AND INVESTIGATIONS

The differential diagnosis includes pseudoporphyria, bullous pemphigoid, bullous impetigo, chronic hand dermatitis, pompholyx, and epidermolysis bullosa acquisita.

Measurement of urine porphyrins is the most sensitive way to diagnose PCT and this also allows for discrimination from pseudoporphyria. Elevation of urine porphyrinogens, with elevated isocoproporphyrins in the stool, is the classic pattern of PCT. Quick examination of the urine under a Wood lamp, after the addition of a few drops of glacial acetic acid, yields a pink–red fluorescence due to the presence of uroporphyrinogens.

Skin biopsy from a blister typically demonstrates a pauci-inflammatory subepidermal blistering disorder. Perivascular porphyrin deposition in the dermis causes 'festooning,' or projections of the papillary dermis into the blister cavity. Reduplication of the basement membrane zone material carried upward into the epidermis leads to visible 'caterpillar bodies.' Still light microscopy cannot allow for confident discrimination of porphyria from pseudoporphyria.

SPECIAL POINTS

Measures that lower hepatic iron stores, such as therapeutic phlebotomy, usually lead to remission in PCT. If phlebotomy is not feasible, antimalarials (such as chloroquine) can be helpful.

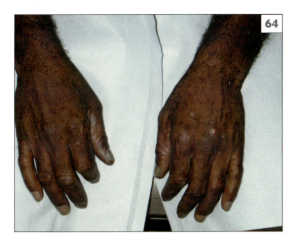

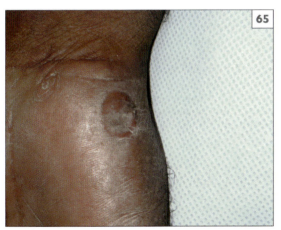

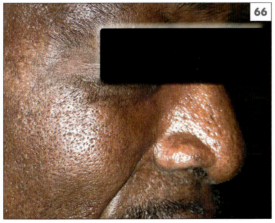

64–66 Porphyria cutanea tarda.

OTHER INFLAMMATORY CONDITIONS

Psoriasis

DEFINITION AND CLINICAL FEATURES

Psoriasis is a papulosquamous inflammatory skin disorder. Despite intense investigation, the cause of psoriasis is not well understood. It would appear that there is a genetic tendency toward psoriasis, but an environmental exposure or 'trigger' is necessary for disease onset. While older references state that psoriasis is a disorder of epidermal proliferation, it is now understood that the disease is chiefly a consequence of aberrant T-cell function.

Classic psoriasis vulgaris presents as erythematous plaques with a distinctive overlying thick silver scale (**67–69**). Psoriasis can develop in any area of the body, but a predilection exists for the posterior scalp, elbows, knees, gluteal cleft, and nails. Common nail findings include minute pitting (**70**), onycholysis, or brown–yellow discolorations of the nail bed itself ('oil staining') (**71**). Pruritus is rarely a substantial complaint in classic psoriasis, and the aesthetic concerns are more apt to concern the patient.

Psoriasis often demonstrates a Köbner response in the skin, which is the appearance of new lesions at the site of trauma. Other associated clinical findings include geographic tongue and arthritis (in 5–30%). Most often, psoriatic arthritis presents as an asymmetric oligoarthritis with involvement of few joints.

Clinical variants of psoriasis include the following:
- Psoriasis vulgaris – classic plaque-type psoriasis (most common).
- Guttate psoriasis – explosive onset of minute ('raindrop-like') psoriatic papules. This variant is more likely to resolve without recurrence than are classic psoriatic plaques. It is most often seen in young patients after a preceding streptococcal infection and it is rare in the elderly.
- Localized pustular psoriasis – also known as pustulosis palmaris et plantaris (pustules of the palms and soles). It creates a waxing and waning pustular eruption on the palmoplantar and acral surfaces.
- Generalized pustular psoriasis (of von Zumbusch) – a rare and fulminant variant associated with generalized erythema and a myriad of small pustules. Patients often experience malaise, fever (up to 104°F), and leukocytosis. This variant may appear after the withdrawal of systemic corticosteroids in a patient with otherwise stable psoriasis and this is the primary contraindication for using oral steroids in psoriasis.

Some medications, including beta-blockers, which are often utilized in the elderly population, can unmask subclinical psoriasis.

EPIDEMIOLOGY

Psoriasis is most common in white people and is rare in black people. Psoriasis is also less common in tropical environments. The incidence of psoriasis in the United States is unknown, but estimates vary from 1% to 3% of the general population. About one-third of patients will report a positive family history of the disease.

DIFFERENTIAL DIAGNOSIS AND INVESTIGATIONS

Psoriasis is most often confused with eczematous conditions. The characteristic presentation in certain bodily locations (the elbows, knees, occipital scalp, and intragluteal area) is common to psoriasis, while many forms of eczema tend to occur in flexural areas (atopic dermatitis) or dependent areas (stasis dermatitis). Examination of other bodily areas, such as the nails, may also provide important corroborating evidence.

A biopsy of a plaque is not always diagnostic of psoriasis, but typically it is helpful in excluding other conditions, such as eczematous conditions (which demonstrate epidermal spongiosis) and hypersensitivity processes (which demonstrate eosinophils) – findings that are unusual in psoriasis and militate against the diagnosis.

SPECIAL POINTS

The treatment of psoriasis is based on the level of disease and symptoms; there are four general categories of treatment:
- Topical treatments – topical steroids, topical vitamin D analogs, anthralin, tar
- Phototherapy – broad- and narrow-band UVB and PUVA, excimer laser
- Oral medications – methotrexate*, cyclosporine, acitretin, fumaric acid (not available in the USA)
- Biologic agents – infliximab*, etanercept*, adalimumab*, ustekinumab*.

*Denotes treatment potentially helpful in psoriatic arthritis.

Patients may need a combination of these therapies and changes throughout their lives based on efficacy and side effects. Since psoriasis is a lifelong condition, a strong therapeutic alliance and considerations of the risks and benefits of multiple options are required.

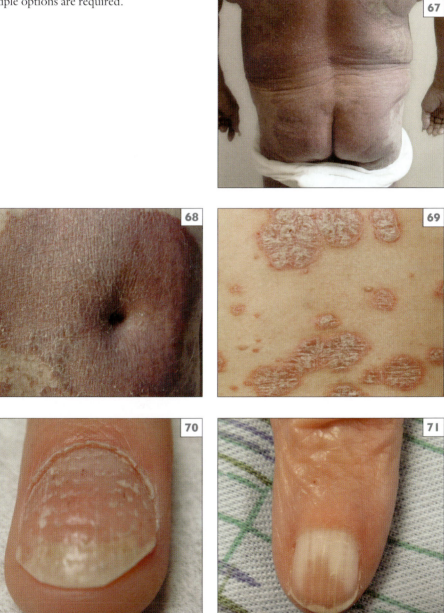

67–71 Psoriasis (**67–69**); psoriasis in nail–pitting (**70**); psoriasis in nail–oil staining (**71**).

Pityriasis rubra pilaris

DEFINITION AND CLINICAL FEATURES

Pityriasis rubra pilaris (PRP) is another chronic papulosquamous disorder of unknown etiology that is much rarer than psoriasis. PRP is characterized by red–orange scaly plaques, palmoplantar keratoderma, and keratotic follicular papules.

PRP often yields an extensive eruption with distinct and interspersed areas of uninvolved skin, referred to as 'islands of sparing' (**72** & **73**). The keratotic papules are often accentuated on the skin of the back of the hands, creating 'nutmeg grater'-looking plaques on the dorsal fingers (**74**). The palmoplantar thickening that produces the keratoderma can be so thick that it interferes with function (**75**).

Pruritus of PRP is often intense, unlike psoriasis. The eruption and the pruritus often develop in a descending fashion, beginning first on the scalp and then slowly progressing downward to involve other areas of the body.

EPIDEMIOLOGY

PRP occurs equally in males and females and involves people of all races. The incidence of PRP has been reported to be about 1 case for every 3,500–5,000 patients presenting to dermatology clinics, and it is not nearly as common as psoriasis.

DIFFERENTIAL DIAGNOSIS AND INVESTIGATIONS

No specific laboratory test exists to confirm the diagnosis of PRP. The diagnosis is usually made through the correlation of clinical and histological findings observed on biopsy. Often early PRP is very difficult to diagnose – hence the adage, 'never be the first to see a case of PRP,' and the condition only becomes diagnostic as the eruption progresses and the palmoplantar keratoderma foments.

SPECIAL POINTS

Treatment of PRP depends on the severity of the disease. Topical steroids and emollients may be helpful in mild or early cases. Systemic retinoids, especially acitretin and isotretinoin, have been used with success. These agents may be easier to

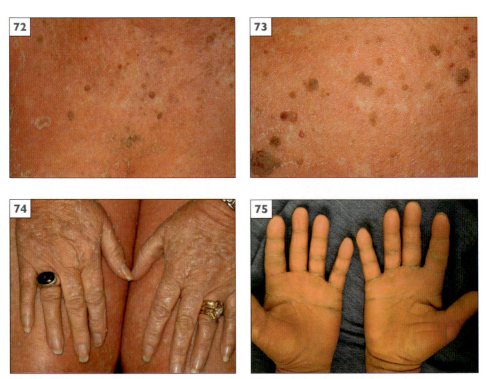

72–74 Pityriasis rubra pilaris.

75 Pityriasis rubra pilari–keratoderma.

use in elderly patients since the prohibitions against pregnancy with their use will usually not be an issue. Second-line agents include methotrexate and systemic immunosuppressives.

Seborrheic dermatitis

DEFINITION AND CLINICAL FEATURES
Seborrheic dermatitis is a papulosquamous disorder that involves characteristic locations on the face, and trunk. The sebum-rich areas of the browline, glabella, nasolabial folds, periauricular area, scalp, and anterior neck and chest are most often involved (**76–78**). The condition produces mild erythema, a subtle greasy yellow scale, dander in the scalp, and a varying degree of pruritus.

While the exact etiology is still disputed, this dermatitis is associated with pathological forms of Pityrosporum organisms called *Malassezia*, as well as aberrant immunological responses to the fungi on the skin. The disease has a tendency to wax and wane over time, and the severity ranges from mild and nearly imperceptible dandruff to exfoliative erythroderma.

EPIDEMIOLOGY
Seborrheic dermatitis affects males slightly more often than females, but up to 10–15% of the population may experience minor forms of the disease in the way of dandruff. The elderly seem particularly affected by seborrheic dermatitis, and it may be aggravated by Parkinson disease and other neurological ailments common to the elderly. Seborrheic dermatitis is also more prevalent and intractable in AIDS.

DIFFERENTIAL DIAGNOSIS AND INVESTIGATIONS
A diagnosis of seborrheic dermatitis is usually made based on a history of waxing and waning severity and by involvement of characteristic areas on physical examination. Sometimes it can be difficult to discriminate between severe seborrheic dermatitis and scalp psoriasis, and often dermatologists refer to such cases as sebopsoriasis, as the distinction does not alter management. The histological findings of seborrheic dermatitis are non-specific and a biopsy is not often of great utility.

SPECIAL POINTS
Antifungal creams or shampoos (such as keto-conazole 2% shampoo used to wash the face and scalp in the shower) are often helpful. Mild topical steroids (including hydrocortisone or desonide creams) can be used as needed on the face and eyebrows. Liquid drop or foam steroid preparations are available for more elegant use on the scalp. It is important to counsel patients about the potential side effects of topical steroids, such as atrophy or telangiectases, since seborrhea is a chronic condition. The steroids should be used only as needed and discontinued if improving. To limit steroid exposure, topical immunomodulators (such as tacrolimus ointment or pimecrolimus cream) are sometimes used.

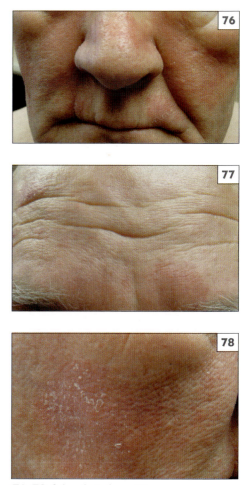

76–78 Seborrheic dermatitis.

Intertrigo

DEFINITION AND CLINICAL FEATURES
Intertrigo is a chronic, irritated condition caused by the confluence of sweat, friction, and overgrowth of skin commensal organisms, usually found in the body folds or in obese patients (**79**). It is most commonly found under the breasts in females, under the pannus in obese patients, and in the inguinal folds. It can be quite irritating or even painful and prevent the patient from being able to walk or exercise normally.

Clinically, it appears as pink or red macerated plaques radiating from the body folds. It often may be moist or feature thick, white scale. Tracking erythema or satellite pustules may be a sign of secondary infection with bacteria or *Candida*.

EPIDEMIOLOGY
Intertrigo is common in adults and more common in females, diabetics, and obese patients. It is very common in the elderly who may be less mobile and have conditions that make routine bathing and drying difficult. It is more common in humid climates or environments.

DIFFERENTIAL DIAGNOSIS AND INVESTIGATIONS
Inverse psoriasis, candidiasis, and irritant contact dermatitis may all produce similar findings and indeed the latter two may be seen commonly with intertrigo.

Routine tests are not needed in the diagnosis of intertrigo, which is typically easily suspected based on history and the physical examination. Swab cultures for bacteria or *Candida* may help if these conditions are suspected.

SPECIAL POINTS
Treatment of intertrigo primarily involves remedying the circumstances that cause it. Weight loss should be encouraged for obese patients. Careful, gentle bathing of the area with a gentle cleanser followed by gentle but complete drying is critical. A hair dryer (on the cool air setting) can be helpful to completely dry under breasts or body folds. Powders (with or without antifungal medications) may help keep the area dry and lubricated. Zinc oxide or other thick, protective pastes can help accomplish the same function. Hydrocortisone is often helpful to decrease irritation and redness.

If there is an underlying condition, such as hyperhidrosis causing excess sweating, it should be treated. Similarly, if secondary infection of the skin with yeast or bacteria is suspected, it should be treated appropriately.

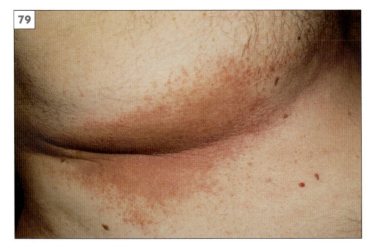

79 Intertrigo.

Asteatotic eczema

DEFINITION AND CLINICAL FEATURES
Simply put, asteatotic eczema is skin that is so dry and xerotic that a frankly eczematous condition results. Due to the fissuring of the skin, it is sometimes called eczema craquelé.

The condition is most often observed on the shins of elderly patients, but it may also occur on the hands and trunk (**80**). Superficial bleeding and fissures occur as the epidermis loses water, and the skin splits enough to disrupt papillary dermal capillaries. The inflammation may also be associated with asymmetric leg edema.

Traditional (or atopic) eczema is less common in elderly patients but may occur and be more widespread and itchy than asteatotic eczema.

Because of the pruritus involved, the patient may scratch at the lesions, leading to further excoriation, bleeding, lichenification, and other secondary features that may obscure the diagnosis.

EPIDEMIOLOGY
Elderly persons with decreased sebaceous and sweat gland activity, and increased xerosis, are particularly predisposed to asteatotic eczema. Similarly, patients on statins for hypercholesterolemia, those who use harsh soaps and degreasing agents, and people bathing with particularly hot water and who do not apply emollients after bathing are more likely to develop the condition. Profound lower extremity edema, more common in the elderly, leads to stretching of the overlying epidermis, which also increases transepidermal water loss and contributes to xerosis.

DIFFERENTIAL DIAGNOSIS AND INVESTIGATIONS
Nummular dermatitis and asteatotic eczema share many similar risk factors and have similar contributory factors. No laboratory investigations are typically necessary and the skin biopsy shows only non-specific histological findings common to all eczematous conditions.

SPECIAL POINTS
Aggressive moisturization is critical in all forms of eczema, but especially in the asteatotic variant. Baths should be short and warm, and soap should be avoided on the affected areas. A thick moisturizer (such as petrolatum) should be applied several times throughout the day. A cool mist humidifier may be helpful if placed in the bedroom in winter months.

When itching or inflammation is marked, topical steroids (ideally in an ointment base) are often used. Antihistamines may also be helpful for itching, but care should be taken since antihistamines that cause drowsiness (such as hydroxyzine and doxepin) may lead to falls or confusion in elderly patients.

For severe cases of eczema, systemic treatment may be needed. UVB phototherapy is often helpful and generally safe in elderly patients. Short courses of systemic steroids are helpful for flares. More aggressive treatment with long-term systemic steroids or immunosuppressive drugs (such as cyclosporine or azathioprine) may be difficult for older patients to tolerate.

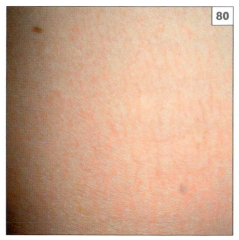

80 Asteatosis.

Lichen planus

DEFINITION AND CLINICAL FEATURES

Lichen planus is another papulosquamous disease of unknown etiology. The disease presents as intensely pruritic, violaceous, polygonal papules that may demonstrate a fine, white, lacy network of lines on the surface ('Wickham striae') (**81–83**). These papules may also coalesce into plaques. Typically the degree of scale is minimal, particularly in respect of other papulosquamous diseases, such as psoriasis.

Mucocutaneous findings of lichen planus are not unusual and include lacy white lesions on the buccal mucosa, and oral ulcerations. The disease may also produce alopecia and nail dystrophy (**84 & 85**).

Thorough examination to discover mucocutaneous involvement is important, because cutaneously limited disease often resolves spontaneously over 1–2 years, but if there is mucosal involvement it often portends a much more prolonged and recalcitrant course.

Lichenoid drug eruptions can often mimic classic lichen planus. At least 83 drugs have been implicated in lichenoid eruptions, with the most common being antimalarials, beta-blockers, furosemide, gold (including that in popular liquors), quinidine, and thiazide diuretics. Many of these agents are often employed in managing disease of the elderly.

EPIDEMIOLOGY

Lichen planus occurs in both sexes and in all racial groups. More than two-thirds of patients are 30–60 years of age, but lichen planus may occur at any age. Long-standing ulcerative lesions of lichen planus in the mouth, particularly in males, have a higher incidence of malignant transformation to squamous cell carcinoma, and vulvar lesions in females may also be associated with this same risk.

DIFFERENTIAL DIAGNOSIS AND INVESTIGATIONS

With the exception of lichenoid drug eruptions, which require a thorough medication history, the diagnosis is usually established based on the clinical appearance and symptoms. A biopsy is often confirmatory. Lichenoid drug eruptions may be impossible to distinguish from classic lichen planus, but often the presence of eosinophils in the dermis on biopsy suggests a drug-induced etiology.

SPECIAL POINTS

Treatment of lichen planus varies with severity and site of the condition. Isolated skin lesions are often treated with topical steroids but courses of systemic steroids may be needed. Phototherapy, both narrow-band UVB and PUVA, may be helpful when steroids alone are not enough. Acitretin, both with and without concomitant phototherapy, is also useful but should be avoided in females of child-bearing potential due to the severe risk of birth defects.

Oral lichen planus can be debilitating, leading to pain and weight loss from inability to eat properly. Topical steroids in a base designed for the oral mucosa (such as triamcinalone compounded in oromucosal paste) may be helpful but often systemic treatments, as listed in the paragraph above, are required.

Some patients with lichen planus also have hepatitis C. A history of risk factors or exposures and a hepatitis C antibody test are appropriate.

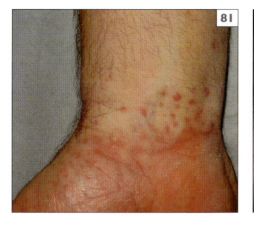
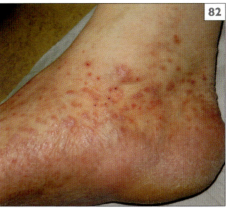
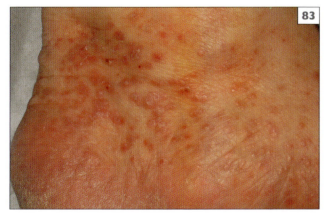

81–85 Lichen planus.

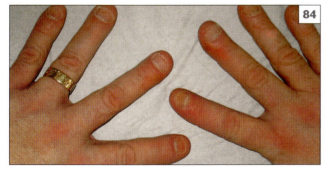
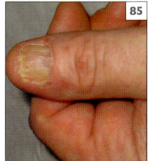

Contact dermatitis

DEFINITION AND CLINICAL FEATURES

Contact dermatitis is a reaction of the skin to an external trigger. It may be truly allergic or caused by irritation, depending on the source. Contact dermatitis is very common in elderly patients, since they are more likely to use medical devices, tapes and bandages, and topical medications.

Allergic contact dermatitis tends to present as eczematous plaques that may be excoriated or secondarily infected. They may be linear or confined to areas of the body exposed to the allergen (**86 & 87**).

Irritant contact dermatitis (**88**) is not a true allergic reaction, but a breakdown of the skin due to an irritating or caustic substance. It tends to be more macerated than allergic dermatitis and is also often found in areas of exposure to the trigger.

EPIDEMIOLOGY

Both allergic and irritant contact dermatitis can be seen at any age but are very common in the elderly patient, although there are few data on their exact prevalence in this population. Elderly patients who still work may be exposed to occupational triggers. Hobbies (such as gardening or woodworking) are another common source of exposure. The use of medical supplies, such as latex gloves, catheters, bandage adhesives, or topical medications, is another common cause and may be seen in patients or their caregivers.

DIFFERENTIAL DIAGNOSIS AND INVESTIGATIONS

It is important to differentiate contact dermatitis from other causes of eczema (such as asteatotic or atopic eczema), since contact dermatitis can often be easily treated by avoiding the cause. A thorough history and physical examination, with special attention to the patient's daily routine and personal care/medical products, can often elicit the diagnosis. Eczematous plaques that are linear or in a specific distribution should also be suspicious for contact dermatitis.

Biopsy will show typical eczematous changes and may not differentiate contact dermatitis. If numerous eosinophils are seen on pathology, it is suspicious for an allergic cause.

Patch testing to the most common allergens is easily accomplished at most dermatology centers and can be helpful when history fails to determine the exact cause. Patch testing may also be helpful if multiple allergens are suspected or in cases of chronic dermatitis of unknown cause.

SPECIAL POINTS

There are many possible causes of contact dermatitis. Among allergic causes, latex, nickel, formaldehyde and its releasers, topical anti-biotics (especially neomycin and bacitracin), and preservatives from personal care products are very common. Phenylenediamine in hair dyes and acrylates in false nails are a common problem for elderly patients. It is important to remember that topical steroids can also cause allergic dermatitis, which can make for a confusing clinical picture since the steroids can both improve and worsen the problem.

Irritant causes also abound in elderly patients. Urine or feces in incontinent patients can easily irritate the skin much as they do in infants. Aggressive hand washing (especially in caregivers or catheterized patients) may strip the hands of their protective oils, leading to irritant dermatitis. Alcohol-based hand sanitizers, cleaning chemicals, and occupational or hobby exposures to solvents are common triggers.

Treatment of allergic contact dermatitis primarily involves identifying and removing the source of the problem. Patch testing may help to identify products to use or avoid. In general, using fewer products and choosing ones that are fragrance free and hypoallergenic is helpful. Commercially available kits allow patients to test metal objects for nickel.

Topical steroids (in an ointment base) are often helpful for allergic dermatitis if the cause cannot be determined. Systemic steroids and UVB phototherapy may also be helpful for recalcitrant cases.

The treatment of irritant dermatitis requires changing behaviors, where possible to avoid the trigger. Gentle cleansers and moisturizers can replace hand sanitizers. Gloves may be helpful when working with cleaners or solvents. For incontinent patients, more frequent changing of diapers and pads, along with barrier creams and powders to absorb moisture, may be needed.

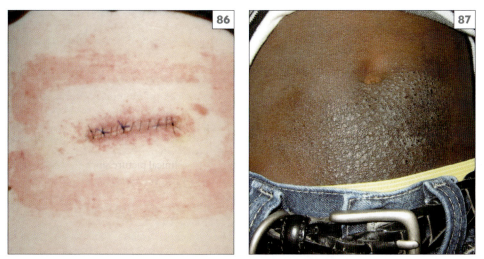

86, 87 Allergic contact dermatitis to adhesive (**85**); allergic contact dermatitis to nickel (**86**).

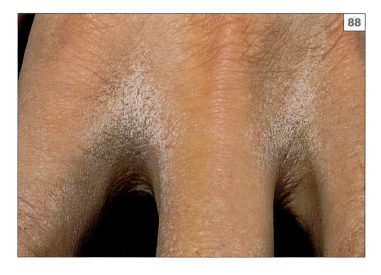

88 Irritant contact dermatitis.

Nummular dermatitis

DEFINITION AND CLINICAL FEATURES

Nummular dermatitis, derived from the Greek word for 'coin,' is a form of eczema that is characterized by the development of round-to-oval erythematous plaques, chiefly on the arms and legs (**89 & 90**). These eczematous plaques may be studded with vesicles early on, and may also have an overlying serous exudate (**91**). Secondary

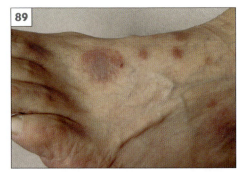

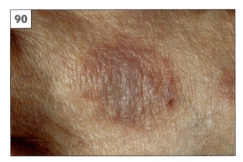

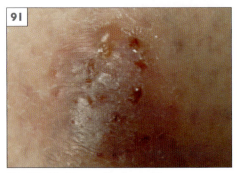

89, 90, 91 Nummular dermatitis.

infection with *Staphylococcus* often occurs within this crust. Pruritus is a common feature.

While the exact cause of the disease is unknown, like asteatotic eczema, the condition is frequently accompanied by xerosis. It is thought that dry and cracking skin may allow for permeation of environmental allergens and induce eczematous changes. One study of elderly patients with nummular dermatitis demonstrated a heightened sensitivity to environmental aeroallergens when compared with age-matched controls.

EPIDEMIOLOGY

The prevalence of nummular dermatitis in the United States is about 2 cases per 1,000 persons. Nummular dermatitis has bimodal age distribution, and it is most common in elderly males in the sixth to seventh decades of life. A smaller peak occurs in the second to third decades of life, among females.

DIFFERENTIAL DIAGNOSIS AND INVESTIGATIONS

The differential diagnosis is established through observation of characteristic lesions in the appropriate clinical setting. A skin biopsy demonstrates only the non-specific histological findings common to all eczematous conditions, although it may be useful to exclude other causes of an annular eruption, such as tinea. Tinea also is more likely to have an active edge with serous crusting, rather than a uniformly eczematous surface. There is no laboratory test for nummular dermatitis.

SPECIAL POINTS

Treatment of nummular eczema usually begins with a gentle bathing regimen (short, warm baths with no soap applied to the affected areas) and topical steroids. Often potent topical steroids (such as clobetasol or fluocinonide ointment) are needed for thicker plaques. Patients should be counseled on the use and long-term side effects of applying potent steroids, including skin atrophy and telangiectases. Monitoring for and treating infection of the plaques (especially with *Staphylococcus aureus*) is important.

Systemic treatments are usually not needed, but a course of systemic steroids or narrow-band UVB phototherapy may be useful in recalcitrant cases or severe flares.

Urticaria (hives)

DEFINITION AND CLINICAL FEATURES

Urticaria is a very common and itchy skin condition defined by 1–2 cm areas of dermal swelling and erythema (weals) (**92**). There should be no scaling and individual lesions always last less than 24 hours (although new ones may arise in that time). It may occur anywhere on the body and has many potential causes, although most cases of chronic urticaria are idiopathic. It may be associated with potentially dangerous swelling in the mouth or throat, especially when allergic in cause.

Acute urticaria is defined as hives present less than 6 weeks. It is often allergic in cause, with insect stings, medications, and foods being common triggers. Associated angioedema of the face and throat is not common, but can lead to difficulty breathing and even death.

Lesions of chronic urticaria appear identical to those in the acute form, but recurrences last longer than 6 weeks and sometimes for many years. The underlying cause can be difficult to find and even extensive testing is often negative. It can be a miserable and frustrating condition for patients.

Dermatographism is a specific form of chronic urticaria seen more commonly in teenage and young patients. It results from physical perturbation of the skin by scratching or rubbing which leads to an urticarial response minutes later. It is not typically associated with underlying disease and often resolves spontaneously after several years.

EPIDEMIOLOGY

Urticaria is extremely common and it is estimated that one in six persons will experience it in their lifetimes. Acute urticaria is generally more common than chronic urticaria. Some forms, such as dermatographism, are less common in elderly patients. Other forms, especially drug induced or hives related to chronic diseases, may be more common in elderly patients.

DIFFERENTIAL DIAGNOSIS AND INVESTIGATIONS

Urticaria is generally clinically classic and can be diagnosed via history and physical examination. If individual lesions last more than 24 hours or leave dyspigmentation, biopsy may be helpful to rule out urticarial vasculitis, a rare condition often associated with connective tissue disease. Urticarial bullous pemphigoid, rare in general but relatively more common in elderly patients, can also confound the diagnosis. Biopsy and immunofluorescence will differentiate.

For acute urticaria, a history of insect bites, new medications, and recent diet can often help elicit the cause. Some of the most common causes include bee stings, antibiotics (especially penicillin and its derivatives), NSAIDs and aspirin, tree nuts, shellfish, and strawberries. Consultation with an allergist may be helpful if the trigger is unclear.

Chronic urticaria may warrant investigation for potential underlying triggers if severe or persistent. A thorough medication history, especially the use of 'as needed' medications, should be undertaken. Common blood tests include CBC, metabolic and liver profile, ESR, ANA, hepatitis B and C serologies, IgE autoantibodies, and *Helicobacter pylori* antibody, but these are often negative and some practitioners do not order any routine blood testing. Stool ova and parasite examination should be ordered if there is clinical cause.

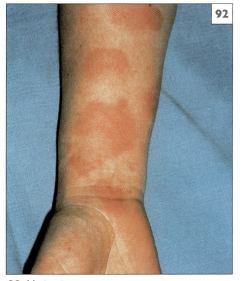

92 Urticaria.

SPECIAL POINTS

The treatment of acute urticaria revolves around removing and avoiding the cause and preventing acute attacks that compromise respiration. A short course of systemic steroids will often clear the hives, although will return if the trigger is not removed. Epinephrine is given urgently in cases of facial or laryngeal edema. A self-injector of epinephrine is often supplied to patients with known severe allergies to stings or foods so that they can administer it immediately if accidentally exposed. These should be used with caution in elderly patients with a history of cardiac disease, since epinephrine can induce tachycardia and even myocardial infarction.

Chronic urticaria can be quite difficult to treat. If an underlying cause cannot be found, treatment usually begins with antihistamines. A non-sedating antihistamine may be helpful in the morning (loratadine or fexofenadine). Sedating antihistamines are often given at bedtime (hydroxyzine or doxepin). These must be used with care in elderly patients, since they can cause confusion and falls. Doxepin also has numerous potential drug interactions.

Systemic steroids will often temporarily relieve a flare of chronic urticaria but are a poor long-term choice due to side effects. More aggressive treatments include cyclosporine, mycophenolate mofetil, azathioprine, and omalizumab, although these can be expensive and difficult to tolerate for elderly patients.

Rosacea

DEFINITION AND CLINICAL FEATURES

Rosacea is a disorder characterized by vaso-motor instability and an acneiform eruption of the face. The spectrum of clinical disease includes varying degrees of baseline erythema, telangiectases, and inflammatory papulopus-tules that resemble common acne (**93–95**). Sometimes there can be involvement of the eyes as well with conjunctivitis, matting, and general irritation. Long-standing rosacea in elderly males may lead to rhinophyma (**96**), or bulbous sebaceous hyperplasia of the soft tissue of the nose.

The cause of rosacea is unknown but certainly environmental triggers appear to be involved in the disease. Patients often note a worsening with sunlight exposure. Ingestions of hot liquids, spicy foods, caffeine, alcohol, and tomatoes are often thought to worsen the condition, as are other harsh environmental exposures, such as prolonged chapping by the wind.

Evidence exists that suggests that these harsh climatic exposures damage cutaneous blood vessels and dermal connective tissue, while the ingestions promote vasomotor instability. Patients with rosacea often characterize themselves as 'flushers' and 'blushers' and there may be proclivity to the disease among such persons.

Some researchers have suggested that *Demodex* species of mites ('oil mites') which normally inhabit human hair follicles in heavily sebaceous areas may play a role in pathogenesis. Furthermore, inconclusive evidence suggests that *Helicobacter pylori* is associated with rosacea, but these studies are plagued by confounding variables such as sex, age, socioeconomic status, and medications.

EPIDEMIOLOGY

Patients with rosacea are disproportionately of northern European, and particularly Celtic, heritage. While exaggerated flushing and blushing may date back to childhood or the early teens, rosacea does not normally present until middle adulthood and it often progresses with age. Rhinophyma is essentially exclusively a manifestation of rosacea seen in elderly males.

DIFFERENTIAL DIAGNOSIS AND INVESTIGATIONS

Rosacea is nearly always diagnosed on clinical grounds. A biopsy is not helpful as it shows non-specific chronic inflammatory infiltrates of the superficial vascular and superficial aspects of the adnexal structures.

SPECIAL POINTS

Rosacea can be treated in a variety of ways. Avoiding triggers, such as sun, heat, emotional stress, spicy food, and alcohol, is often helpful. Sunscreen with a spectrum to protect against UVA and UVB, along with a hat, should be used daily.

Topical treatments include metronidazole gel and azelaic acid. If these are not enough, systemic antibiotics such as doxycycline or minocycline are often used. Since rosacea is a chronic condition, these treatments must often be continued indefinitely.

Many older patients have had rosacea for many years and so may have more prominent erythema on the cheeks and telangiectases. These are often best treated, if bothersome, by laser or light-based modalities, such as pulsed dye laser or intense pulsed light. Rhinophyma can be treated with destructive modalities such as a hot-wire loop or ablative CO_2 laser.

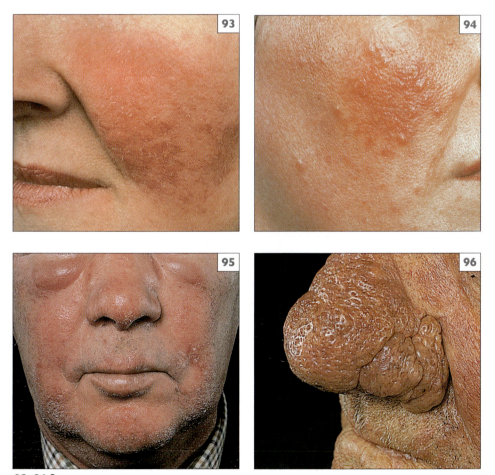

93–96 Rosacea.

Lichen sclerosus

DEFINITION AND CLINICAL FEATURES

Lichen sclerosus is a chronic inflammatory dermatosis, likely of autoimmune etiology, that presents with white plaques on the body with associated epidermal atrophy. Common lichen sclerosus occurs on the perineum of females (**97**), but also on the glans penis of males, where it is called balanitis xerotica obliterans (**98**). However, extragenital presentations occur as well. In large series, genital presentations, both vulvar and penile, outnumber extragenital reports by more than 5:1.

Besides the atrophy and possible stricture of the introitus (females) or urethral meatus (males), the plaques are often intensely pruritic. An increased risk of squamous cell carcinoma may exist with long-standing vulvar disease, but the precise degree of this risk and the involvement of any cofactors are not well defined.

EPIDEMIOLOGY

Lichen sclerosus is a rare disease, but the exact incidence within the population is unknown. Females are affected far more often than are males, with a ratio of about 6:1. About 85% of cases occur in adults.

DIFFERENTIAL DIAGNOSIS AND INVESTIGATIONS

Because of the intense pruritus, some cases of lichen sclerosus can be confused with lichen simplex chronicus occurring in the genitalia (pruritus vulvae). A biopsy is a convenient way to make the diagnosis as there are diagnostic histological findings and this will also exclude other concerns such as tinea, vulvar cancers, and even coexisting squamous cell carcinoma as a manifestation of long-standing lichen sclerosus.

SPECIAL POINTS

Lichen sclerosus can be very painful and cause dyspareunia. Topical steroids are typically the first line of treatment and high-potency steroids (such as clobetasol ointment) are usually required. Since high-potency steroids are not typically used on sensitive skin, such as the genitals, it is important to instruct the patient on use and monitor for atrophy. Vitamin D analogs, such as calcipotriene (calcipotriol) ointment, may be helpful for long-term treatment since they are steroid free. UVA-1 phototherapy is not widely available but is found in some larger dermatological centers; it has been shown to be helpful in sclerosing conditions, including lichen sclerosus.

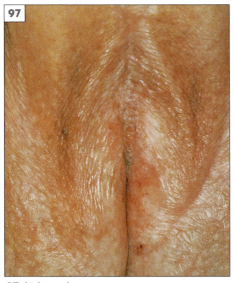

97 Lichen sclerosus.

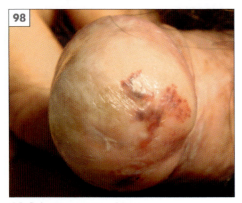

98 Balanitis xerotica obliterans.

Neurodermatitis/Prurigo nodularis/Lichen simplex chronicus

DEFINITION AND CLINICAL FEATURES
Prurigo nodularis and lichen simplex chronicus are related forms of neurodermatitis. Both conditions result from the chronic manipulation of the skin secondary to pruritus or other perceived dysesthesias.

Prurigo nodularis usually presents as multiple, intensely pruritic, excoriated papules and nodules erupting on the extensor surfaces of the limbs, and other reachable areas of the body. There is often an unusual and unnatural appearance to the lesions (**99 & 100**). Lichen simplex chronicus is also characterized by chronic manipulation, but it tends to form single or multiple acanthotic plaques, with overlying hyperkeratosis and some hyperpigmentation.

Chronic trauma and mechanical irritation of the skin causes thickening called lichenification. Repetitive rubbing, scratching, and touching, whether occurring with one's hands or with another object, results in these changes.

Occasionally, prurigo nodularis or lichen simplex chronicus has an underlying trigger, such as folliculitis, insect bites, or long-standing low-grade eczematous conditions or metabolic disturbances (liver or kidney failure), but quickly the secondary features of manipulation supersede as the dominant pathological process.

EPIDEMIOLOGY
Lichen simplex chronicus and prurigo nodularis may occur at any age, but the conditions most often occur in middle-aged and older persons.

DIFFERENTIAL DIAGNOSIS AND INVESTIGATIONS
Prurigo nodularis occurring in the elderly may be concerning for non-melanoma skin cancer, as the areas of sun exposure and accessibility for manipulation overlap significantly. Similarly, lichen simplex chronicus may be confused with psoriasis or any long-standing eczematous condition. Skin biopsy for histological examination and/or cultures may be indicated to exclude skin cancer or infection, or psoriasis, or to suggest a primary eczematous disorder.

SPECIAL POINTS
Avoiding rubbing or scratching is critical to the improvement of neurodermatoses, but can be very difficult. In the elderly patient the condition may be further complicated by dry skin, difficulty in applying moisturizer, or dementia.

Topical or intralesional steroids can help decrease itching. Antihistamines also help with itching but must be used with caution in a geriatric population, since they can cause drowsiness, which may lead to falls and confusion. Covering the affected area or using a distraction (such as squeezing a racquetball when the urge to itch strikes) may prevent picking.

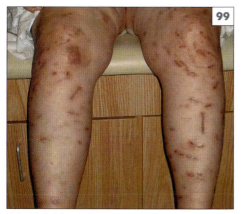
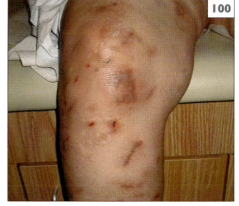

99, 100 Neurodermatitis.

Chondrodermatitis nodularis chronica helicis

DEFINITION AND CLINICAL FEATURES

Chondrodermatitis nodularis chronica helicis (CNCH) is a painful reactive dermatosis that occurs as a result of chronic pressure applied to the skin, soft tissue, and cartilage of the helix or antihelix of the ear.

While the exact pathogenesis of the disorder is unknown, most authorities believe that it is caused by prolonged and excessive pressure on the sun-damaged skin and soft tissue of the ear that possesses little subcutaneous tissue for padding. Dermal inflammation, edema, and necrosis result, and, ultimately, this leads to perichondritis.

Clinically, the result is a painful, hyperkeratotic papule on the helix or antihelix of the ear (**101**). Sometimes there is central ulceration and crusting. The right ear is more often involved than the left in most large series. Sleeping exclusively on one side of the body often results in disease on that ear.

EPIDEMIOLOGY

CNCH more often affects middle-aged or older males, and this is thought to be related to hairstyles in males that result in greater sun damage to the ears, but cases in females also transpire. Furthermore, it is thought that the condition is more common on the right ear because of the vast predominance of right-handed individuals who utilize the right hand to hold telephone headsets and other apparatus that come in contact with the ear.

DIFFERENTIAL DIAGNOSIS AND INVESTIGATIONS

Because the lesions occur on the sun-exposed skin of middle-aged to elderly individuals the chief concern is discriminating CNCH from non-melanoma skin cancer, including basal cell carcinoma and squamous cell carcinoma. A biopsy is generally performed when there is sufficient need to exclude a malignant process.

SPECIAL POINTS

Avoidance of repeated ear trauma is critical in treatment. Special 'ear pillows' with a hole cut for the ear are available. If possible, the patient should sleep on the opposite side from the affected ear.

Intralesional or topical steroids may help temporarily with pain and inflammation. If persistent, the lesion can be surgically excised.

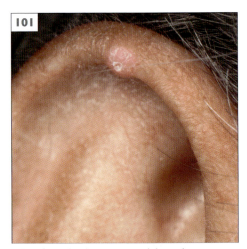

101 Chondrodermatitis nodularis chronica helicis.

Grover disease

DEFINITION AND CLINICAL FEATURES

Grover disease, also known as transient acantholytic dermatosis, is a benign, self-limited disorder that results in a pruritic, papular eruption on the trunk (**102–104**). The exact cause of the disease is unknown, although there is often an association with a preceding heat exposure and/or prolonged sweating. While severe cases may also involve the proximal extremities, the scalp and distal extremities are almost always spared.

Interestingly, while all patients with Grover disease experience pruritus, the clinical appearance does not always correlate with the symptomatology. For example, some patients with very limited cutaneous disease may complain of intractable itching, while others with many papular lesions have vastly more limited symptoms.

While a significant number of patients with Grover disease will complain of a preceding fever (that leads to overheating and sweating) there are no systemic manifestations of the disease.

EPIDEMIOLOGY

Grover disease usually affects middle-aged to elderly white males, although it may be seen in other races. The ratio of affected males to females exceeds 3:1.

DIFFERENTIAL DIAGNOSIS AND INVESTIGATIONS

Grover disease should be distinguished from other papular and intensely pruritic disorders such as a papular urticaria, miliaria, and scabies. A skin biopsy of Grover disease shows the histological finding of acantholytic dyskeratosis.

SPECIAL POINTS

Treatment of Grover disease is based on the level of symptoms. For milder cases or in older patients where systemic treatment carries more risk, topical steroids are often helpful. A lotion vehicle (such as triamcinolone lotion) can be especially helpful since it is easy to spread over larger areas.

For more severe cases, tetracycline, phototherapy, and systemic retinoids (such as acitretin or isotretinoin) may be helpful.

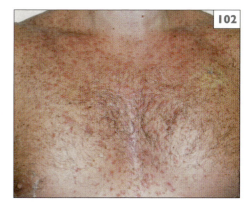

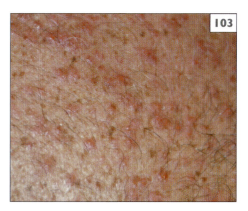

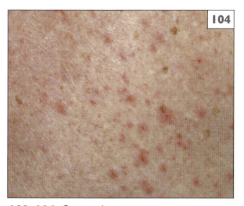

102–104 Grover disease.

Erythema annulare centrifugum

DEFINITION AND CLINICAL FEATURES

Erythema annulare centrifugum (EAC) is reactive figurate erythema. It is characterized by annular, erythematous lesions with an internal edge ('trailing edge') of light scale (**105 & 106**). Lesions are usually 2–5 cm in diameter, and, while pruritus may be present, it is generally a lesser feature than that of other annular conditions, particularly tinea.

The etiology of the disorder is unknown, but the condition is thought to represent a hypersensitivity reaction to a variety of agents, including drugs, arthropod bites, infections (bacterial, mycobacterial, viral, fungal, filarial), ingestions (blue cheese), endocrine disturbances (pregnancy), and even rarely malignancy.

EPIDEMIOLOGY

The exact incidence of EAC is unknown but certainly the condition is uncommon. A case series from England estimated the incidence to be approximately 1 case per 100,000 persons in the population per year. It has been reported in a wide variety of patients from infancy to the ninth decade of life.

DIFFERENTIAL DIAGNOSIS AND INVESTIGATIONS

To exclude tinea, a KOH skin scraping may be performed. As some forms of lupus may be in the differential diagnosis, an ANA and/or ENA test may be helpful when this appears to be a diagnostic possibility. Other tests, such as endocrinological assessments should be based on the history, review of systems, and the clinical examination.

A skin biopsy may be helpful in confirming a diagnosis of EAC but the histological pattern of a superficial and deep perivascular lymphocytic infiltrate is not exclusive to this disease process, and it may be of greater utility in ruling out other conditions such as lupus or tinea.

SPECIAL POINTS

EAC often resolves without treatment but topical steroids may be used symptomatically. If tinea is present, it should be treated, as the condition may resolve once the fungal infection improves.

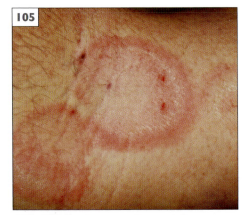 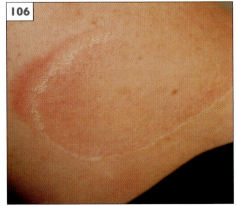

105, 106 Erythema annulare centrifugum.

Erythema nodosum

DEFINITION AND CLINICAL FEATURES

Erythema nodosum is a nodular, erythematous eruption usually limited to the anterior pretibial surfaces of the lower legs. It is presumed to be a hypersensitivity reaction and may occur in association with several systemic diseases or drug therapies, or it may be idiopathic.

The lesions begin as erythematous, tender nodules on the shins (**107 & 108**). As the process lies deep in the subcutis, the borders at the surface are poorly defined. Typically the lesions vary from 2 cm to 6 cm in size. During the first week, the lesions become tense, hard, and painful, while during the second week they may become more fluctuant. Yet the lesions of erythema nodosum do not suppurate or ulcerate. Aching legs, swelling ankles, and even arthralgias may also be noticed.

EPIDEMIOLOGY

Females are affected by erythema nodosum more often than males. The female:male ratio is about 4:1. The condition is most common in young adults aged 18–34 years, but it may occur at any point in life including the elderly.

DIFFERENTIAL DIAGNOSIS AND INVESTIGATIONS

Erythema nodosum can be confused with a deep-seated infection or possibly erythema induratum, another reactive panniculitis, although this latter condition is more common on the posterior leg in the region of the calf. To confirm the diagnosis, it is important to perform a deep biopsy (to fat), as a superficial biopsy will provide no intelligible information.

Because of a strong association with streptococci, a throat culture is often included as part of the initial workup for erythema nodosum. Antistreptolysin O titers may be elevated, but normal values do not exclude streptococcal infection. Additional laboratory testing should be based on the history and clinical examination.

SPECIAL POINTS

Lesions of erythema nodosum can be quite painful and treatment is often required. First-line treatment includes examining for and treating underlying causes, elevation, and NSAIDs. The last should be used with caution in elderly patients due to the increased risk of bleeding.

Systemic steroids and SSKI can be helpful in recalcitrant cases but require close monitoring in the elderly patient due to the risk of side effects.

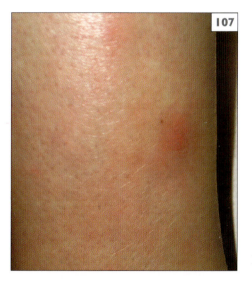

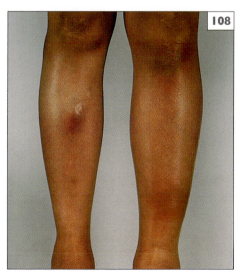

107, 108 Erythema nodosum.

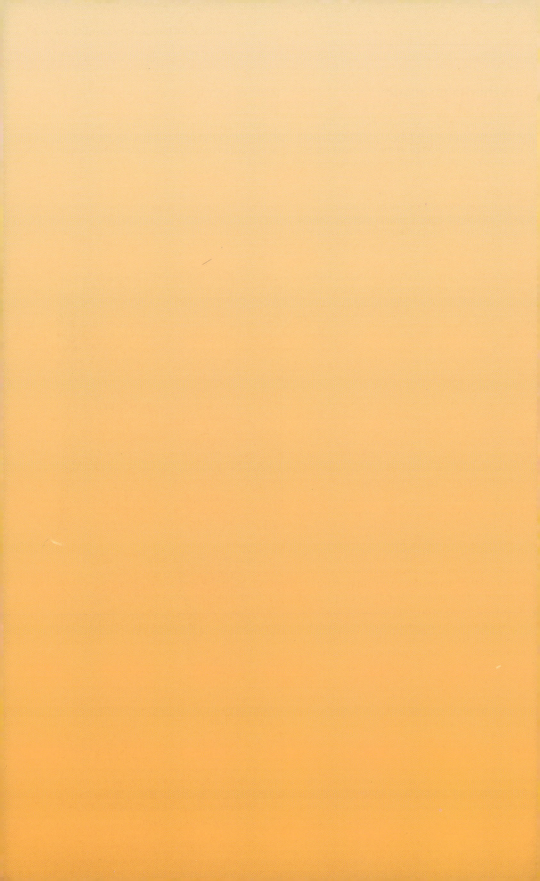

PART 3

Neoplasms of the skin

- **Malignant**

- **Benign**

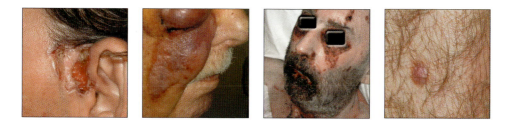

MALIGNANT

Basal cell carcinoma

DEFINITION AND CLINICAL FEATURES

Basal cell carcinoma (BCC) is a slow-growing, locally destructive, malignant neoplasm of basal keratinocytes. It is the most common cancer in humans and particularly common in the elderly. BCC, for practical purposes, does not metastasize and poses a local, but generally not systemic, threat.

BCC has many distinct clinical presentations. The most common type, nodular BCC, presents as a pearly papule with a rolled edge, often with telangiectases (**109–111**). It is sometimes ulcerated and can present simply as a non-healing wound (**112 & 113**). Nodular BCC usually presents on sun-exposed skin, especially the face and ears. Pigmented variants exist (**114 & 115**).

Superficial BCC presents as a thin plaque with a sharply defined border and it can be very large (**116**). Superficial variants may appear scaly, but other types of BCC are generally not scaly.

Morpheaform BCC exhibits scar tissue intermixed with the malignant basal cells and can clinically mimic a scar. These lesions tend to be more infiltrative and more difficult to treat than other types.

There is a pigmented form of BCC which occurs in darker-skinned individuals. It is usually similar to the nodular variant except for its blue to black coloration.

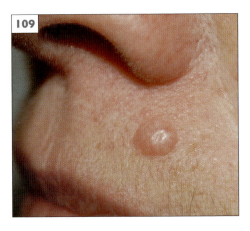

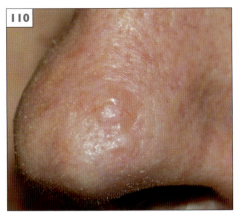

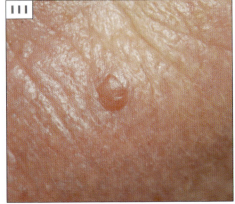

109–111 Basal cell carcinoma.

EPIDEMIOLOGY

BCC is overwhelmingly caused by sun exposure, often routine exposure over many years. Ionizing radiation, pre-existing benign neoplasms (such as nevus sebaceous), and certain genetic syndromes (such as basal cell nevus syndrome and xeroderma pigmentosum) can also predispose to BCC.

BCC is common in general, more common in males than females, and more frequently seen in older patients. It is most common in fair-skinned patients and much rarer in darkly pigmented persons. Rates of BCC rise the closer a patient lives to the equator.

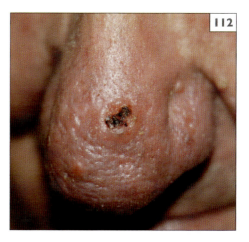

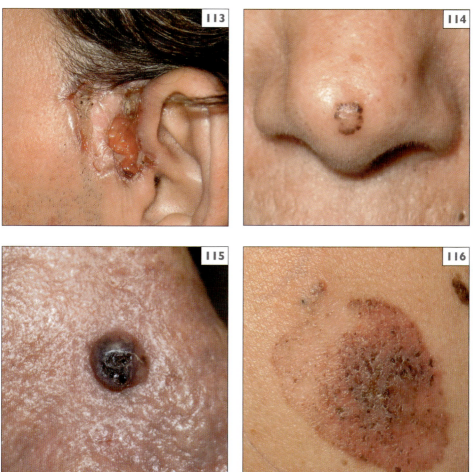

112–116 Ulcerated basal cell carcinoma (112, 113); pigmented basal cell carcinoma (114, 115); superficial basal cell carcinoma (116).

DIFFERENTIAL DIAGNOSIS AND INVESTIGATIONS

The differential diagnosis includes other types of skin cancer, especially squamous cell carcinoma. Benign entities, such as neurofibroma, seborrheic keratosis, or a fibrous papule, may mimic BCC. Any type of irritated benign skin lesion on sun-exposed skin, especially if there is extensive bleeding or crusting, may cause confusion. The pigmented variant is sometimes confused with melanocytic lesions (such as a nevus or melanoma).

Diagnosis is usually clinical supported by biopsy, which is definitive. Suspicious lesions should always be sampled, both to confirm the diagnosis and to rule out more aggressive types of skin cancer. Although lesions are sometimes treated without biopsy if they are clinically typical, biopsy before treatment is generally preferred, as some subtypes (especially morpheaform examples) may require more aggressive treatment.

Microscopically, BCC shows a proliferation of basaloid cells in the epidermis and dermis. Morpheaform variant often shows admixed scar and may exhibit infiltrative malignant cells. Pigmented examples often exhibit significant brown or black pigment within the abnormal basal cells.

SPECIAL POINTS

Since BCC is almost never fatal, a holistic approach to the elderly patient and treatment should be adopted. Although surgical excision or destruction is often the treatment of choice, topical and other less aggressive therapies are commonly used in very elderly or infirm patients. Treatment should be customized to a patient's health status, age, and other comorbidities.

Curettage and electrodessication are especially popular in elderly patients because they are quick to perform, effective, and do not require suturing. Excision with histological confirmation of complete excision is also frequently performed. Mohs micrographic surgery is frequently used for large lesions (especially >2 cm), lesions with infiltrative or morpheaform behavior, or lesions on areas where tissue conservation is paramount (face, ears, hands).

Non-surgical alternatives also exist. Cryotherapy has been used for many years to treat BCC and may be easier on an elderly patient than surgery. Imiquimod and fluorouracil creams are sometimes used for superficial BCC. Radiotherapy is also quite effective and can be better tolerated by older patients with comorbidities.

Actinic keratosis

DEFINITION AND CLINICAL FEATURES

Actinic keratosis (also called solar keratosis) is a sun-induced precursor to squamous cell carcinoma. There is debate about whether actinic keratosis is a precancerous lesion or simply the earliest form of squamous cell carcinoma. These lesions are extremely common in elderly patients, especially those with a long history of sun exposure.

Actinic keratoses occur usually on sun-exposed skin as adherent, rough, thin, flesh-colored, or erythematous papules. They tend to occur on the bald scalp, face, ears, neck, dorsal forearms, and hands (**117–119**). Lesions can be asymptomatic or painful, often described as a 'burr' or 'pin' in the skin. At times, they may be felt by the examiner as a rough papule, even when they are difficult to see. Patients frequently have multiple lesions.

Similar changes on the lips (usually the lower lip) are referred to as actinic cheilitis.

EPIDEMIOLOGY

Actinic keratoses tend to be more common in males, persons who have lived in sunny climates, and older patients. They are extremely rare in dark-skinned patients unless an underlying genetic syndrome is at work.

The vast majority occur due to chronic sun exposure. They more rarely occur due to ionizing radiation exposure, arsenic exposure (such as with pesticide-contaminated drinking water), or certain predisposing genetic syndromes (such as xeroderma pigmentosum).

DIFFERENTIAL DIAGNOSIS AND INVESTIGATIONS

The most important differential diagnosis is an early squamous cell carcinoma, due to its different treatment needs. Since actinic keratosis and squamous cell carcinoma are made of the same cells (malignant keratinocytes), they can sometimes be very difficult to distinguish. Superficial basal cell carcinoma can also mimic actinic keratosis.

Benign lesions, such as benign lichenoid keratosis, irritated seborrheic keratosis, or warts (especially flat warts) can also be confused with actinic keratoses.

Diagnosis is usually clinical and lesions are often treated without biopsy. Biopsy is sometimes necessary, however, to distinguish from squamous cell carcinoma or other non-melanoma skin cancers.

Microscopically, actinic keratosis demonstrates atypical keratinocytes that do not extend to the full thickness of the epidermis (once they fill the epidermis, they are designated squamous cell carcinoma *in situ*). They can be superficially thick (hypertrophic actinic keratosis) or be at the base of a cutaneous horn.

SPECIAL POINTS
Although only a portion of actinic keratoses progresses to squamous cell carcinoma, it is impossible to predict which will transform and they always need to be treated. Liquid nitrogen applied via a specially designed canister or a cotton-tipped applicator is the most common approach. Application of aminolevulinic acid followed by photodynamic therapy is also effective. Topical therapy with fluorouracil or imiquimod cream can achieve a field effect if a patient has numerous lesions. Chemical peels with Jessner solution or trichloroacetic acid can also be effective for treating numerous lesions simultaneously.

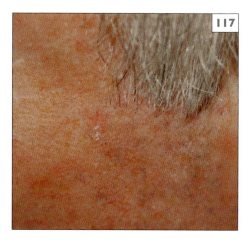

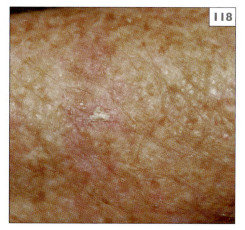

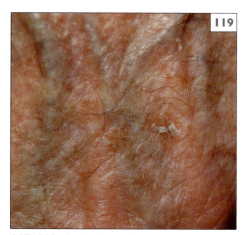

117–119 Actinic keratosis.

Squamous cell carcinoma

DEFINITION AND CLINICAL FEATURES

Squamous cell carcinoma (SCC) is a malignant neoplasm of epidermal keratinocytes, usually induced by the sun. Although early lesions are usually treated with local surgery, SCC does have the potential to metastasize. It is the second most common cancer (after basal cell carcinoma) in humans and is especially common in elderly patients.

SCC presents as a poorly defined, expanding, erythematous, and sometimes ulcerated plaque or nodule, usually on sun-exposed skin (**120**). Overlying scale or crusting is common. A cutaneous horn may be present overlying the lesion (**121–123**). The surrounding skin often shows actinic keratoses or signs of chronic sun damage. Superficial variants of SCC *in situ* (Bowen disease) also exist (**124**).

EPIDEMIOLOGY

SCC of the skin is common and more frequently seen in older patients due to their increased levels of lifetime sun exposure.

SCC is usually induced by chronic sun exposure and less commonly by arsenic exposure, radiation exposure, photochemotherapy (such as PUVA), or genetic syndromes (such as xeroderma pigmentosum). Fair-skinned individuals are at increased risk since their skin offers less protection from the sun.

Scars, especially from sites of burns or radiation exposure, can degenerate into SCC. Chronic immunosuppression is also a risk factor and SCC is frequently seen in transplant recipients. Sites of chronic, long-term inflammation, as is seen in discoid lupus erythematous or chronic ulcers, are also at increased risk. Smoking is a risk factor for lip lesions.

DIFFERENTIAL DIAGNOSIS AND INVESTIGATIONS

Other forms of non-melanoma skin cancer, such as basal cell carcinoma, must be distinguished. An advanced actinic keratosis can also be mistaken for an early SCC, since they are on the same clinical continuum. Chronic infections, especially with fungi or atypical mycobacteria, or other types of chronic inflammation can mimic SCC.

Clinical suspicion is raised by a thorough examination with good lighting and a hand lens. A biopsy to confirm the diagnosis and evaluate for worrisome features (such as invasion or poor differentiation) is required if SCC is suspected. Although multiple biopsy techniques can diagnose SCC, one that provides a broad breadth of the neoplasm is preferred. Excisional, incisional, saucerization, and shave biopsies can all be useful.

Full-thickness atypia of squamous cells that is confined to the epidermis, without invasion, is referred to as SCC *in situ* (Bowen disease). When the malignant cells penetrate the dermis, it is called invasive SCC. Tumors are also sometimes categorized by level of depth of invasion differentiation, with deeper and more poorly differentiated tumors behaving more aggressively.

SPECIAL POINTS

Surgical excision, either traditional excision or Mohs micrographic surgery, is preferred so histological margins can be evaluated. In elderly patients too infirm to undergo surgery, options include cryotherapy, curettage, and electrodessication, and topical imiquimod or fluorouracil cream. These techniques are generally more successful with smaller and non-invasive lesions. Photodynamic therapy has also been tried for superficial lesions.

The local lymph node basins should always be examined to check for metastasis. A CT scan or sentinel lymph node biopsy can be performed to look for subclinical metastasis in large or poorly differentiated lesions. The rate of metastasis is especially high for lesions on the ears, lips, and genitals.

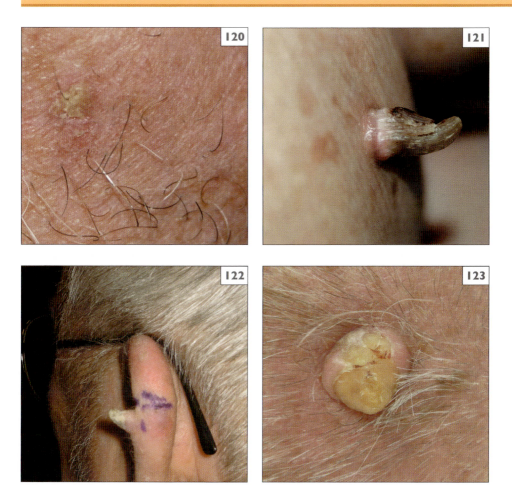

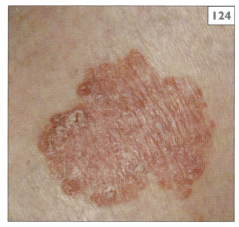

120–124 Squamous cell carcinoma.

Keratoacanthoma

DEFINITION AND CLINICAL FEATURES

A rapidly growing, volcanic neoplasm, keratoa-canthomas usually appear on sun-exposed skin (**125–127**). A keratoacanthoma can grow astonishingly quickly and sometimes resolve without treatment. Some others, however, progress to squamous cell carcinoma, so treatment is usually advised.

Keratoacanthomata almost always arise over days or weeks. They present as a solitary, dome-shaped, sharply circumscribed papulonodule, often in the setting of actinic damage. They are quite exophytic and can become painful or easily traumatized.

EPIDEMIOLOGY

Keratoacanthomas are most common in fair-skinned patients of middle age or older. Although they can resemble squamous cell carcinoma under the microscope, they are clinically distinct due to their rapid growth and potential for spontaneous involution. Their exact cause is unknown although chronic sun damage is thought to play a role.

Rarely, multiple lesions occurring at once (eruptive keratoacanthoma) can occur. Eruptive keratoacanthomas have sometimes been associated with internal malignancy.

DIFFERENTIAL DIAGNOSIS AND INVESTIGATIONS

The rapid growth and sharp demarcation of keratoacanthoma can help to clinically distinguish it from squamous cell carcinoma or basal cell carcinoma. Although clinical examination alone can usually diagnose a keratoacanthoma, a biopsy is warranted to assess for squamous cell carcinoma.

Microscopically, atypical squamous epithelium is seen in a sharply demarcated, cup-like pattern with a central core or crust. Lesions are usually well circumscribed. Some dermatopathologists distinguish between a classic (benign) kerato-canthoma and a more malignant-appearing squamous cell carcinoma, keratoacanthoma type.

SPECIAL POINTS

Keratoacanthomata are often treated via surgical excision. This technique allows for pathological confirmation of clear margins, which can be especially important in cases where transformation to squamous cell carcinoma is suspected.

Destructive techniques, such as cryotherapy, and curettage and electrodessication, are also frequently employed. Intralesional methotrexate is effective and there are some reports of success with intralesional triamcinolone. These methods are especially useful in very elderly or infirm patients, who may poorly tolerate traditional excision.

True keratoacanthomas generally resolve without treatment after several months. Watchful waiting is not much employed, however, due to the rapid growth of these lesions and possibility of squamous cell carcinoma.

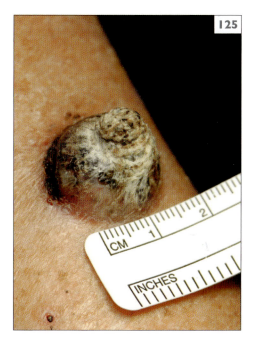

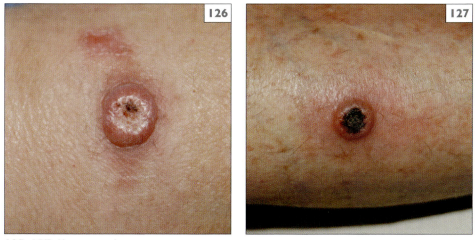

125–127 Keratoacanthoma.

Malignant melanoma

DEFINITION AND CLINICAL FEATURES

Melanoma is the most dangerous common form of skin cancer. A malignant tumor of pigment-generating melanocytes, melanoma is caused, in part, by UV exposure. It has a high potential for metastasis if not detected and removed early and a poor prognosis once it has spread outside the skin. It can occur in patients of any age, but is less common in children.

Melanoma usually presents as an irregularly shaped or bordered, pigmented macule or papule (**128 & 129**). They are often asymmetric, have scalloped borders, and feature multiple colors in the same lesion. Nodular lesions afford an ominous prognosis, but do not involve a diagnostic dilemma (**130**). Although they commonly occur on sun-exposed skin, they can occur anywhere on the body. Melanomas also occur less commonly in the nail unit, retina, and gastrointestinal tract. Amelanotic (non-pigmented) melanoma can also occur, which can be very difficult to diagnose clinically, as it can mimic squamous cell carcinoma or benign neoplasms. Metastatic lesions may be widely dispersed or agminated (**131**).

The lentigo maligna subtype is slow growing and almost always found on the face or neck of elderly patients. It is usually a large, hyperpigmented macule, at times mimicking a large lentigo or seborrheic keratosis (**132**). Indeed, a biopsy is often needed to discriminate between these conditions.

Although darker-skinned patients are less likely to develop melanoma, they tend to have more aggressive lesions, often arising on the hands or feet.

EPIDEMIOLOGY

Melanoma is most frequently caused by chronic exposure to the sun. Previous sunburns each sequentially increase the risk of melanoma. Fair-skinned individuals are also at increased risk, although melanoma can occur in any skin type. Genetic predisposition to melanoma is also possible. A family history of melanoma and/or a personal or family history of atypical (dysplastic) nevi puts a patient at increased risk.

DIFFERENTIAL DIAGNOSIS AND INVESTIGATIONS

Seborrheic keratoses, benign or dysplastic nevi, angiokeratoma or other vascular tumors, and pigmented basal cell carcinoma can all mimic melanoma. The amelanotic subtype is especially difficult to diagnose, since the traditional ABCD criteria used to assess pigmented lesions may not apply.

A biopsy is critical for suspected or potential melanomas. It is important that the biopsy encompass the full depth of the lesion, since Breslow depth (the depth of invasion of the

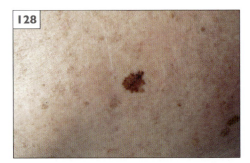

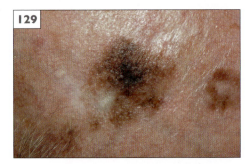

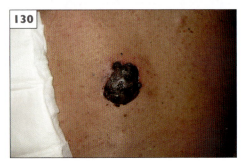

128–130 Melanoma.

atypical melanocytes) is a critical piece of prognostic information and cannot be determined if the lesion is transected. An excisional biopsy, saucerization biopsy, or punch biopsy (if the lesion is small) is, therefore, preferable for a suspected melanoma. For extremely large lesions (such as lentigo maligna) or infirm patients, an incisional biopsy of the darkest or most irregular portion can be performed. It should be noted, however, that the darkest portion does not always correlate to the most atypical and the diagnosis may be missed if only part of the lesion is sampled.

Microscopically, melanoma exhibits atypical melanocytes, often in nests. If confined to the epidermis, it is called melanoma *in situ*. Invasive melanomas are measured for Breslow depth (from the deepest part of the tumor to the granular layer of the epidermis) and Clark level (determined by how much of the dermis is filled with tumor). Breslow depth is directly correlated to survival, with deeper lesions being more dangerous.

SPECIAL POINTS

Surgical therapy with adequate margins is the mainstay of melanoma treatment. For very elderly or infirm patients, in whom surgery is not feasible, cryotherapy and topical imiquimod have been utilized. These latter are recommended only in unusual cases, since even a small amount of residual melanoma can lead to metastasis and death.

A clinical lymph node examination should be performed on all patients with melanoma. Sentinel lymph node biopsies are frequently performed, usually on lesions between 1 mm and 4 mm of Breslow depth. CT or, increasingly, PET scanning is also used to detect metastasis.

The treatment of metastatic melanoma is difficult and requires an experienced oncologist. Radiation and traditional chemotherapy are generally ineffective. Interferon-alfa is sometimes used, but can be difficult for the elderly patient to tolerate. Trials of immunological therapies, such as interleukin-2 injections and vaccines against melanoma components, are ongoing.

Patients with melanoma should have careful screening for subsequent primary melanomas. A full-skin examination every 4 months for the first 2 years after diagnosis is recommended.

A team approach is often needed in melanoma treatment, requiring a partnership of dermatologist or primary care physician (for diagnosis and subsequent screening), surgical oncologist, and medical oncologist.

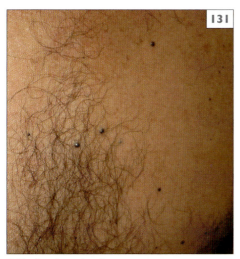

131 Agminated melanoma metastases.

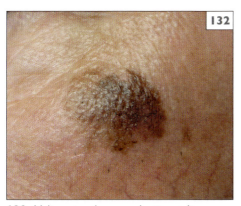

132 Malignant melanoma – lentigo maligna subtype.

Sebaceous carcinoma

DEFINITION AND CLINICAL FEATURES

Sebaceous carcinoma is a rare and potentially dangerous cancer of the sebaceous glands. Although it is rare in general, it is most commonly found in elderly patients.

Sebaceous carcinoma usually presents as a slowly growing, 1–4 mm, firm, yellow nodule on the face or neck (**133 & 134**), and especially the skin near the eyes or eyelids. They often destroy nearby normal structures such as hair follicles or eyelashes.

EPIDEMIOLOGY

Sebaceous carcinoma occurs primarily on the head and neck of elderly patients and is especially common near the eyes. Radiation exposure is associated in some, but not most, cases. The etiology of sebaceous carcinoma is unknown.

DIFFERENTIAL DIAGNOSIS AND INVESTIGATIONS

Sebaceous carcinoma is frequently mistaken for a chalazion on the eyelid. It can also mimic other forms of non-melanoma skin cancer, such as basal cell or squamous cell carcinoma (**135**).

Given the potentially dangerous behavior of sebaceous carcinoma, biopsy is warranted if any clinical suspicion is present. It may also be found unexpectedly on biopsy of a suspected basal cell or squamous cell carcinoma from the face.

Microscopically, cells of varying sebaceous differentiation show an infiltrative pattern both at the lateral edges and the deep margin of the neoplasm. These cells are often full of lipids made by the malformed sebaceous glands.

SPECIAL POINTS

Aggressive treatment is warranted since a sebaceous carcinoma can metastasize. Mohs micrographic surgery is often helpful to define its infiltrative borders on excision. Lymph nodes should be clinically evaluated at each visit. Metastasis to regional lymph nodes and distant metastases are possible. Consultation with an oncologist may be necessary for further radiological workup and adjunctive treatment.

Although rare, Muir–Torre syndrome can cause both sebaceous and colorectal carcinomas. Gastrointestinal workup (colonoscopy, barium enema, and so on) is warranted in patients with sebaceous carcinoma.

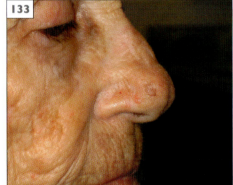

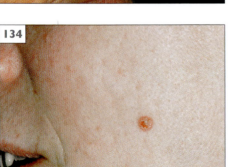

133, 134 Sebaceous carcinoma.

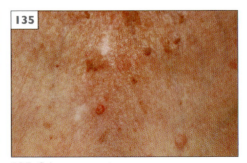

135 Sebaceous carcinoma.

Angiosarcoma

DEFINITION AND CLINICAL FEATURES

Angiosarcoma is an aggressive, multifocal, vascular malignancy, often seen on the head and neck of elderly patients.

Angiosarcoma often appears as a large, poorly defined, red plaque with nodules on the head or neck. Sites of chronic lymphedema can also give rise to angiosarcoma.

EPIDEMIOLOGY

Angiosarcoma is most common in the elderly. It is more common in males than in females by a 2:1 ratio.

Most angiosarcoma is idiopathic. It can, however, occur at sites of post-surgical lymphedema (Stewart–Treves syndrome) or primary lymphedema. Early angiosarcoma may mimic benign vascular tumors such as a hemangioma or pyogenic granuloma (**136**), appearing as a papule or nodule. Later-stage angiosarcoma often presents as any erythematous to violaceous plaque (**137 & 138**).

DIFFERENTIAL DIAGNOSIS AND INVESTIGATIONS

Although it can be clinically suspected when large, erythematous nodules appear on the head or neck of an elderly patient, biopsy is required for diagnosis.

Microscopically, poorly defined and often large collections of vascular spaces are seen, usually lined with atypical endothelial cells demonstrating frequent abnormal mitoses.

SPECIAL POINTS

Angiosarcoma is difficult to treat. A wide local excision is recommended, but such surgery is often disfiguring and sometimes impossible. Radiotherapy may also be used as an adjunct to surgery. Consultation with experienced medical and surgical oncologists is necessary.

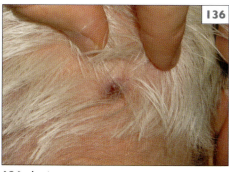

136 Angiosarcoma.

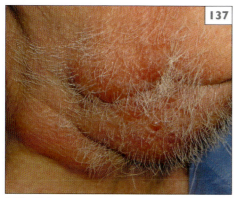

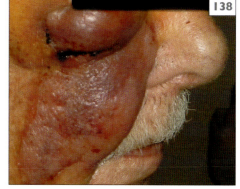

137, 138 Angiosarcoma.

Kaposi sarcoma

DEFINITION AND CLINICAL FEATURES

Kaposi sarcoma is a slow-growing neoplasm most commonly now seen in association with late-stage HIV and AIDS. The traditional (also called classic or endemic Kaposi sarcoma) form, which was present for centuries before HIV, occurs on the lower legs of elderly patients, especially those of Mediterranean or Eastern European descent.

Traditional Kaposi sarcoma appears on the extremities (classically the lower legs) of elderly patients, especially males. It begins as erythematous or violaceous patches that progress to plaques and/or nodules (**139 & 140**). Lymphedema or distal pitting edema may also be present.

The HIV-associated form occurs in younger patients and can occur anywhere on the body. This form may involve the face or trunk more frequently than traditional Kaposi sarcoma.

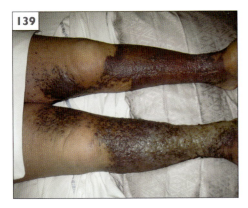

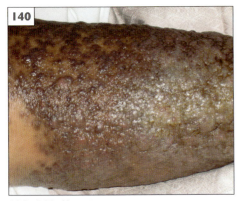

139, 140 Kaposi sarcoma.

EPIDEMIOLOGY

Kaposi sarcoma occurs in two distinct populations: elderly patients (with endemic Kaposi sarcoma) and patients with AIDS.

Kaposi sarcoma (both the traditional and HIV-associated types) is believed to arise from infection with HHV-8. It is thought that relative immunosuppression (from either AIDS or age) allows the virus to proliferate and cause the sarcoma. Transplant recipients are also at risk due to iatrogenic immunosuppression. The endemic form is more common in males.

Some believe that Kaposi sarcoma is not a true malignancy but rather a widespread inflammatory reaction to proliferating HHV-8.

DIFFERENTIAL DIAGNOSIS AND INVESTIGATIONS

Kaposi sarcoma must be distinguished from other vascular neoplasms or purpura. Other dermal inflammatory conditions, such as granuloma annulare or stasis dermatitis, may mimic Kaposi sarcoma. A biopsy is required for diagnosis. If suspected or confirmed, HIV testing is warranted.

Microscopically, numerous slit-like vascular channels are seen in all types of Kaposi sarcoma. Scattered mast cells, erythrocytes, and iron pigment may also be seen in the surrounding dermis.

SPECIAL POINTS

Nodules of Kaposi sarcoma can be excised surgically. Local destruction is also often effective, especially via cryotherapy. Radiotherapy can be effective to treat larger fields. Intralesional (vinblastine, bleomycin) and systemic chemotherapy are also used.

Endemic Kaposi sarcoma often has a slow and indolent course. Depending on the age and health status of the patient, conservative measures may be the most tolerable.

HIV-associated Kaposi sarcoma requires aggressive treatment to raise the CD4+ cell count of the patient. The sudden appearance of Kaposi sarcoma often coincides with a drop in CD4+ cell count. Successful treatment of advanced HIV with a corresponding increase in CD4+ cells will often cause the sarcoma to improve.

Cutaneous B-cell lymphoma

DEFINITION AND CLINICAL FEATURES
Cutaneous B-cell lymphoma (CBCL) is a malignancy of atypical lymphocytes. It may either occur originally in the skin (primary B-cell lymphoma) or spread to the skin from underlying nodal disease. CBCL generally appears as a deeply red or purple nodule or series of nodules in the skin.

EPIDEMIOLOGY
There are many different types of both primary and secondary CBCL. Any of these types may occur in the elderly, although primary cutaneous large B-cell lymphoma of the leg is especially common in elderly females and bodes a poor prognosis (**141**).

DIFFERENTIAL DIAGNOSIS AND INVESTIGATIONS
CBCL, especially small lesions, may be difficult to distinguish from other nodules in the skin including other vascular neoplasms and cysts.

If CBCL is suspected, a biopsy of the lesion is necessary. If confirmed, a clinical lymph node examination and CBC are warranted. Depending on the type of lymphoma, consultation with a medical oncologist and a CT scan in conjunction with a bone marrow biopsy to look for underlying disease may be necessary.

Microscopically, CBCL show numerous, closely packed and atypical lymphocytes. These cells should stain positive for B-cell markers, such as CD20.

SPECIAL POINTS
Although uncommon, CBCL may occur in the elderly and can be highly variable in both aggressiveness and response to treatment based on the type of lymphoma present. A thorough workup for underlying disease and consultation with an experienced medical oncologist is necessary.

141 B-cell lymphoma of the leg.

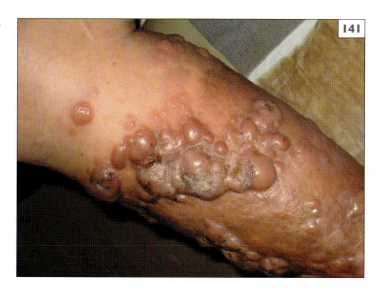

141

Cutaneous T-cell lymphoma

DEFINITION AND CLINICAL FEATURES

Cutaneous T-cell lymphoma (CTCL) (also called mycosis fungoides) is an uncommon, slowly progressive skin infiltration of malignant T lymphocytes. Although it can be progressive and fatal, most cases are indolent and conservative therapy is often the safest option.

CTCL can be very subtle clinically and mimic many other chronic dermatoses. It most frequently consists of chronic, erythematous patches and thin plaques with or without scale on the trunk and extremities (**142–144**). It may be most visible on sun-protected sites, such as the buttocks. Patients may have had the skin eruption for years or decades without major symptoms or a diagnosis.

A hypopigmented variant is seen in darker-skinned patients (**145 & 146**). Patches and plaques are still present, but are usually hypopigmented and scaly. Again, the lesions may have been present for years without a specific diagnosis.

Thicker plaques, nodular lesions, erythroderma, and lymphadenopathy can all be found in more advanced cases.

EPIDEMIOLOGY

CTCL is more common in males than females. Although it can occur in young patients, it is more common after age 50.

Most CTCL is idiopathic. Viral causes, such as human T-cell lymphotropic virus also exist. Some believe that several previously described chronic skin conditions (such as parapsoriasis) are simply early examples of CTCL.

DIFFERENTIAL DIAGNOSIS AND INVESTIGATIONS

The differential diagnosis is extensive, since CTCL can mimic other chronic conditions. Psoriasis, eczema, extensive tinea, and chronic drug reactions can all appear clinically similar. The hypopigmented variant in dark-skinned patients can be mistaken for tinea versicolor, pityriasis alba, and chronic vitiligo. CTCL should be considered in any long-term, chronic

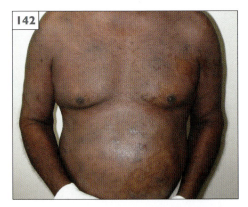

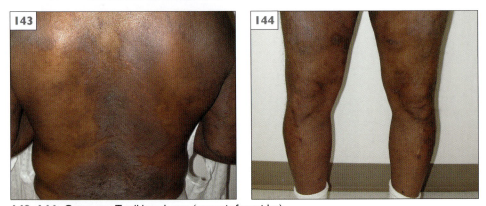

142–144 Cutaneous T-cell lymphoma (mycosis fungoides).

skin eruption without a clear diagnosis or appropriate response to treatment.

Multiple biopsies are often required as the histopathological findings can be subtle. T-cell gene rearrangement studies of both skin and blood can be helpful, although clonality of T cells in the skin can be seen in other, benign conditions. Lymph node biopsy can be performed, if necessary. A CBC with a manual examination for Sézary cells is recommended. Sézary cells are large lymphocytes with large, cerebriform nuclei and occur in Sézary syndrome, the leukemic form of CTCL, which portends a poorer prognosis. LDH levels may also be increased. Testing for human T-cell lymphotropic virus is recommended, especially if the patient is from an endemic area. A CT scan may be helpful if more advanced disease is suspected to identify subclinical or internal lymphadenopathy.

Microscopically, CTCL demonstrates abnormal lymphocytes in the epidermis (epidermotropism) and in microabscesses (Pautrier microabscesses). It can be difficult to distinguish from other lichenoid or lymphocytic reactions, especially if the T cells are only mildly atypical, and repeated biopsies or T-cell gene rearrangement studies are often needed.

SPECIAL POINTS

Management of CTCL depends primarily on the level of disease.

Early stage disease (in which only the skin is affected) is best managed conservatively. Phototherapy (UVB or PUVA) is often quite helpful. Topical therapies include steroids, nitrogen mustard, and bexarotene gel.

More advanced disease (including nodular skin disease, lymph node, or systemic involvement) requires systemic therapy, often under the care of a multidisciplinary team including an experienced medical oncologist. Systemic retinoids (especially bexarotene and sometimes in combination with phototherapy), methotrexate, photopheresis, and chemotherapy have all been utilized.

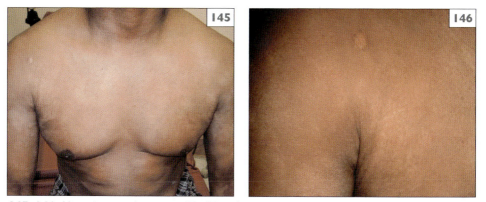

145, 146 Hypopigmented cutaneous T-cell lymphoma.

Metastatic tumors and paraneoplastic syndromes

DEFINITION AND CLINICAL FEATURES

Elderly patients are at increased risk for cancers of many types and these may metastasize to the skin. The skin may be one of many organs affected by metastasis or it can be the initial sign of an internal malignancy. Some internal cancers can also cause skin findings without direct spread, the so-called paraneoplastic syndromes.

Metastasis can present in a variety of different ways. The scalp is a common site of metastases due the large amount of blood that is supplied to it. Certainly, spread to the skin may also be from local extension (such as breast cancer to the overlying skin of the chest), lymphatic spread, or hematological spread.

Certain tumors maintain clinical features of the originating organ. For example, vascular-appearing metastases (red, friable, bleeding) often originate from vascular organs such as the thyroid, kidneys, blood (lymphoma and leukemia), or liver (**147**). Metastases from glandular malignancies (such as breast or colon carcinoma) may exhibit abnormal glandular structures in the skin. Metastases from melanoma are often pigmented or black. Melanoma is also capable of producing bizarre discoloration of normal body fluids when widely metastatic, such as melanuria (black urine when the bladder is heavily involved) (**148**) or black phlegm.

Paraneoplastic syndromes can be more variable. They can include blistering disorders, such as paraneoplastic pemphigus often seen in or near the mouth (**149**), keratoderma, thickening of the palms and soles seen with malignancies of the aerodigestive tract, and discrete nodules, such as Sweet syndrome seen with acute myelogenous leukemia. Since internal malignancies are especially common in the elderly, any unusual, persistent, or treatment-resistant skin condition in an elderly patient should at least be considered for a potential underlying neoplasm.

EPIDEMIOLOGY

Paraneoplastic syndromes vary in occurrence with the underlying cancers that cause them. They are rare overall since they occur in only a small fraction of patients with a given cancer. Skin metastases also vary with the type of cancer involved, but melanoma and breast cancer are specifically prone to skin involvement.

DIFFERENTIAL DIAGNOSIS AND INVESTIGATIONS

Skin metastases often appear as atypical or unusual neoplasms. Although they may be few or solitary, they can also appear as very numerous monomorphic lesions. They may be difficult to distinguish, especially when solitary, from other benign and malignant skin neoplasms. In an elderly patient, any unusual growth should be biopsied.

If a lesion suspicious for metastasis is biopsied in a patient without a known history of internal malignancy, special stains may be used to try to identify the organ or origin and direct the search for internal malignancy. If the lesion is too poorly differentiated for typing, an extensive workup for internal malignancy is usually required.

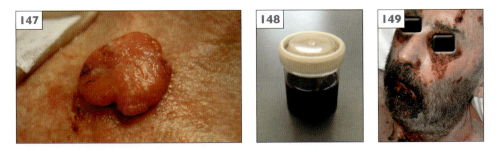

147–149 Metastatic renal cell carcinoma to the skin (**147**); melanuria from systemic melanoma (**148**); paraneoplastic pemphigus (**149**).

SPECIAL POINTS

Treatment of metastasis to the skin or paraneo-plastic syndromes centers on treating the under-lying malignancy, if possible. Skin-directed therapy generally works only to minimize skin symptoms while the patient is undergoing chemotherapy, radiation, or other treatments to target the underlying disease.

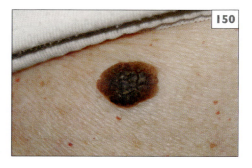

BENIGN

Seborrheic keratosis

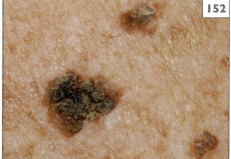

DEFINITION AND CLINICAL FEATURES

Seborrheic keratoses are common, benign keratinocytic neoplasms that occur in adults. Although completely benign, their potential for growth, pigmentation, and crusting can lead to confusion with more concerning diagnoses such as melanoma or squamous cell carcinoma. They are often of cosmetic concern to patients, especially when present on the face, neck, or upper extremities.

Seborrheic keratoses present as warty, flesh-colored to hyperpigmented macules, papules, and small plaques, usually on the scalp, face, neck, trunk, or proximal extremities (**150 & 151**). They often have sharply defined borders and a 'stuck on' appearance. These lesions can become irritated from friction or minor trauma leading to erythema, crusting, and bleeding. Very dark or black lesions are not unusual and may be clinically difficult to distin-guish from melanocytic lesions (**152**). Conversely, lesions on the lower legs, particu-larly the ankle area, take on a whiter hue, and are often called 'stucco keratoses' (**153**).

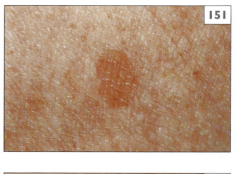

150–152 Seborrheic keratosis.

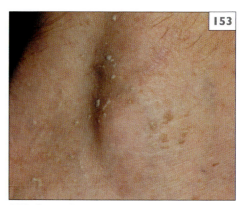

153 Stucco keratoses.

The sudden appearance of numerous seborrheic keratoses in a patient with few or no previous lesions is called the sign of Leser–Trélat and may herald a variety of internal malignancies (**154**).

EPIDEMIOLOGY
The etiology of seborrheic keratoses is poorly understood. They tend to occur in adults and older patients tend to have more of them than younger ones. There is great individual variability between patients: from single lesions to hundreds. Multiple theories have been proposed as to the cause of these lesions, including genetic mutations in local cells and viral causes. Although they sometimes occur in sun-exposed areas, they are generally not thought to be caused by UV radiation.

Dermatosis papulosa nigra is thought to be a variant of seborrheic keratoses and presents with hyperpigmented and often pedunculated papules on the face and neck of dark-skinned patients.

DIFFERENTIAL DIAGNOSIS AND INVESTIGATIONS
Although the diagnosis of seborrheic keratosis is often clinically clear, the lesions can simulate many other lesions at times. Deeply or irregularly pigmented seborrheic keratosis may mimic melanocytic lesions such as dysplastic nevi and melanoma. Crusted or thick lesions may mimic squamous cell carcinoma or pigmented basal cell carcinoma. Macular or thin papular lesions may mimic solar lentigines. Concerning or unusual lesions warrant a biopsy for confirmation.

These lesions are extremely common in elderly patients and diagnosis is usually clinical. Suspicious or unusual lesions, however, should always be sampled to rule out skin cancer. A dermatoscope can be clinically useful for visualizing the horn cysts common to many seborrheic keratoses.

Microscopically, seborrheic keratosis shows a sharply defined, benign-appearing proliferation of basaloid cells with papillomatosis in the epidermis. Small cysts forming within the lesion (horn cysts) are common.

SPECIAL POINTS
Seborrheic keratoses generally do not require treatment. Irritated or bothersome lesions can be removed with liquid nitrogen, curettage, electrosurgery, or shave biopsy. As with all benign lesions, the risk of scarring should be considered prior to treatment. Seborrheic keratoses are not pre-malignant. There is no known way to prevent future lesions.

Patients with sudden-onset, numerous seborrheic keratoses should undergo age- and symptom-appropriate cancer screening.

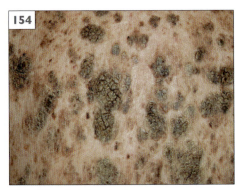

154 Seborrheic keratosis.

Sebaceous hyperplasia

DEFINITION AND CLINICAL FEATURES
Lesions of sebaceous hyperplasia are very common benign overgrowths of sebaceous (oil) glands, generally found on the face of adults with more lesions as the patient grows older. They are completely benign but sometimes cosmetically bothersome.

Sebaceous hyperplasias are commonly found on the face of adult patients (**155 & 156**). They present as 1–3 mm yellow papules, often with a central umbilication (**157**), and may resemble somewhat a basal cell carcinoma. They may have an 'opening flower' appearance. Larger lesions are possible but less common. There is a wide variety in the number of lesions present, from one to dozens. They are typically persistent over time unless removed.

EPIDEMIOLOGY
Sebaceous hyperplasia is a benign overgrowth of a normal structure. It is noticed by the patient or practitioner when the gland becomes large enough to be visible to the naked eye. They tend to be more common in patients with oily complexions. Since they are persistent, elderly patients may accumulate many of them.

DIFFERENTIAL DIAGNOSIS AND INVESTIGATIONS
Since they occur on the face, sebaceous hyperplasia (especially large or atypical lesions) can be confused with basal cell carcinoma and other types of benign or malignant adnexal neoplasms.

These lesions are extremely common in elderly patients and diagnosis is usually clinical. Suspicious lesions, however, should be sampled to rule out skin cancer.

Microscopically, sebaceous hyperplasia shows enlarged but benign sebaceous lobules opening to a central ostium.

SPECIAL POINTS
Sebaceous hyperplasia generally does not require treatment. Large or cosmetically bothersome lesions can be destroyed with light electrosurgery, cryotherapy, acid application (such as trichloroacetic acid), or surgical removal. As with all benign lesions, the risk of scarring should be considered prior to treatment.

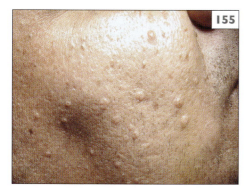

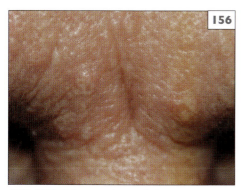

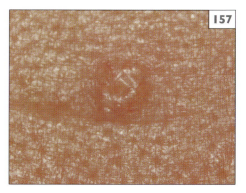

155–157 Sebaceous hyperplasia.

Angioma (cherry angioma)

DEFINITION AND CLINICAL FEATURES

Cherry angiomas are extremely common and benign overgrowths of blood vessels in the skin. They typically appear bright red and well defined, although darker or deeper lesions can sometimes be present. They are especially common in elderly populations and were formerly called senile angiomas.

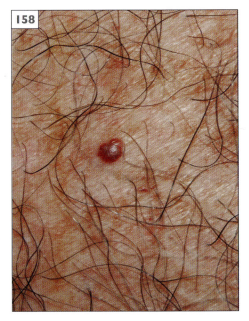

Cherry angiomas present as pinpoint to 5 mm bright or dark red papules on the scalp, face, trunk, and proximal extremities (**158 & 159**). Larger variants are possible. Many patients have multiple lesions (sometimes hundreds), especially on the trunk. Once a cherry angioma arises, it is persistent unless removed. They are, therefore, extremely common in older patients.

EPIDEMIOLOGY

Cherry angiomas are extremely common in both males and females. They tend to first arise in adulthood and become more numerous with age. They frequently begin or become more numerous during pregnancy. There is no known specific environmental or infectious cause of these lesions.

DIFFERENTIAL DIAGNOSIS AND INVESTIGATIONS

Deeper, darker, or purple lesions can be confused with pigmented or melanocytic lesions. Other small vascular lesions (such as angiokeratoma or pyogenic granuloma) may appear similar.

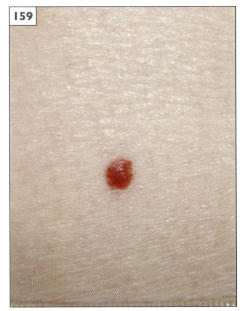

Diagnosis is usually made clinically. Unusual lesions should be biopsied to confirm the diagnosis.

Microscopically, cherry angiomas exhibit sharply circumscribed collections of normal-appearing and somewhat dilated venules.

SPECIAL POINTS

These lesions generally do not require treatment. For cosmetic removal, treatment with a pulsed dye or diode laser is often quite helpful. Light electrocautery can also be effective. If the diagnosis is in doubt a shave or punch biopsy should be helpful.

158, 159 Angioma.

Angiokeratoma

DEFINITION AND CLINICAL FEATURES

Angiokeratomas are benign vascular neoplasms, commonly found in patients over 40 years of age. They can be solitary or occur in large numbers on the scrotum or vulva (angiokeratomas of Fordyce). Although benign, they are important to recognize, as they are often dark in appearance and can mimic melanocytic lesions.

Solitary angiokeratomas appear as single, red–black or red–blue papules (**160**). Angiokeratomas of Fordyce appear as multiple lesions on or near the genitals. These patients may present concerned about a sexually transmitted disease.

EPIDEMIOLOGY

There is no known cause of angiokeratomas, although lesions tend to begin in adulthood and become more numerous with age. Individual lesions tend to be persistent unless removed.

DIFFERENTIAL DIAGNOSIS AND INVESTIGATIONS

Darker angiokeratomas can be confused with melanocytic lesions, either benign or malignant. Lesions on the genitals can be mistaken for genital warts.

Diagnosis is usually made clinically. Dermoscopy may be useful in differentiating them from melanocytic lesions. Suspicious or unusual lesions should be biopsied.

Microscopically, angiokeratomas feature dilated and thin-walled vessels sometimes with thrombosis and overlying parakeratosis.

SPECIAL POINTS

These lesions generally require no treatment. Solitary lesions can be excised with a small surgical excision or a punch biopsy. Multiple lesions can be treated with electrocautery, cryotherapy, or laser treatment (pulsed dye or 532 nm KTP laser).

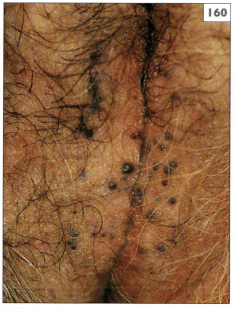

160 Angiokeratoma.

Milium

DEFINITION AND CLINICAL FEATURES

Milia are very common small cysts that occur on the face, especially around the eyes. Although they are benign, they are often of concern to patients either cosmetically or as potential skin cancers. They are commonly found in elderly patients. Sun exposure is a risk factor for milia, especially on the face.

Milia present as 1–2 mm domed white (or sometimes yellow) papules, often near the eyes or elsewhere on the face (**161 & 162**). Unlike the closed comedones (whiteheads) of acne, they typically do not resolve with time. Solitary lesions are common but multiple, eruptive, and plaque-like lesions are also seen. Milia can also be seen in or near scars.

EPIDEMIOLOGY

Milia are extremely common. Although they can occur at any age, they are common in elderly patients. As cumulative lifetime sun damage increases, so does the risk of milia. Rarely, certain blistering disorders (such as porphyria cutanea tarda) can cause multiple milia. There is no known environmental or infectious cause of these lesions.

DIFFERENTIAL DIAGNOSIS AND INVESTIGATIONS

Patients often confuse milia with lesions of acne (closed comedones). They can also mimic pustules, such as those seen in folliculitis. Small lesions of sebaceous hyperplasia can also appear similar.

Diagnosis is generally made clinically. Extraction or biopsy of suspicious lesions to confirm diagnosis is rarely necessary.

Microscopically, milia are essentially tiny and superficial epidermoid cysts with a thin cyst cavity lined with keratin debris.

SPECIAL POINTS

Milia are benign and generally do not require treatment. Individual lesions can be opened with a lancet or scalpel and extracted with a comedone extractor.

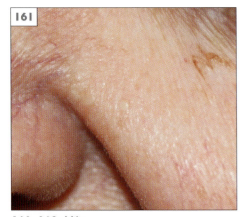

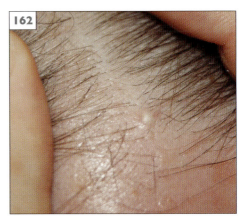

161, 162 Milia.

Skin tags (acrochordons)

DEFINITION AND CLINICAL FEATURES

Skin tags (sometimes called acrochordons) are extremely common, benign, pedunculated neoplasms usually seen at body folds. They are frequently bothersome to patients, both cosmetically and due to irritation from friction (such as from jewelry, shirt collars, or skin folds), or minor trauma. Since lesions do not spontaneously resolve, elderly patients sometimes have accumulated many.

Skin tags present as one to many, 1–4 mm, pedunculated, soft, flesh-colored papules, most commonly on the eyelids, neck, axillae, inframammary skin, and groin (**163 & 164**). Large lesions (even up to several centimeters) are possible but less common.

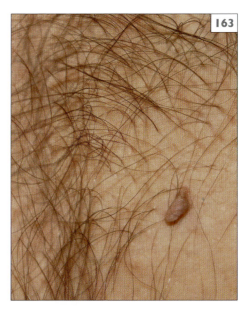

EPIDEMIOLOGY

The exact etiology of skin tags is unknown. They seem to be more common in obese patients and patients with adult-onset diabetes and/or acanthosis nigricans. They are extremely common in elderly patients. There is no known specific environmental or infectious cause of these lesions.

DIFFERENTIAL DIAGNOSIS AND INVESTIGATIONS

Pedunculated verrucas or seborrheic keratoses can sometimes mimic skin tags. Other pedunculated examples of benign neoplasms (such as neurofibromas) can appear similar. Thrombosed or very irritated lesions may appear darker and mimic melanocytic lesions.

The diagnosis is almost always made clinically. Unusual lesions should be biopsied. Microscopically, skin tags show pedunculated hyperplastic and distended epidermis, sometimes with underlying vascular or lymphatic structures seen in larger examples.

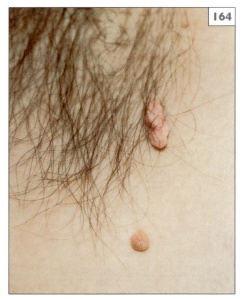

SPECIAL POINTS

For typical lesions, no treatment is required. For irritated or cosmetically bothersome lesions, removal via scissor excision (with local anesthesia for larger lesions) or cryotherapy is effective. Cryotherapy can cause hypopigmentation in darker-skinned patients, who should be warned about this potential complication prior to treatment.

163, 164 Skin tags.

Epidermoid cyst

DEFINITION AND CLINICAL FEATURES

Epidermoid cysts are very common, benign neoplasms that occur in adults. They are often bothersome to patients due to their size, repeated irritation, or the foul-smelling discharge they produce. Many patients have several lesions and some have many. The occasionally used term 'sebaceous cyst' is inaccurate, since these lesions do not arise from sebaceous glands.

Epidermoid cysts generally present as 3–30 mm, domed nodules, often with an overlying punctum connecting them to the surface of the skin (**165 & 166**). Pressure can sometimes cause the expression of cheesy, foul-smelling keratin. Epidermoid cysts most commonly occur on the trunk and proximal extremities, but may be seen on the face, neck, and lower extremities. Most lesions appear bland but irritated examples can be quite swollen, erythematous, and tender. Formerly irritated or recurrent lesions may exhibit surrounding scarring.

EPIDEMIOLOGY

Epidermoid cysts are more common in males than females and can occur from teenage years to the very elderly. As they are usually persistent if not removed, they are extremely common in elderly patients.

The exact cause of epidermoid cysts is unknown. One theory holds that epidermal components introduced into the dermis by a minor trauma cause these lesions to form. There is no known specific environmental or infectious cause of these lesions.

DIFFERENTIAL DIAGNOSIS AND INVESTIGATIONS

Other types of cysts, such as milia near the eyes or pilar cysts on the scalp (**167**) can clinically mimic epidermoid cysts. Lipomas are usually deeper and more poorly defined. Inflammatory conditions that produce nodules, such as panniculitis, may mimic inflamed lesions. Very inflamed cysts may mimic an acute abscess.

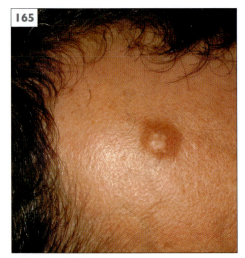

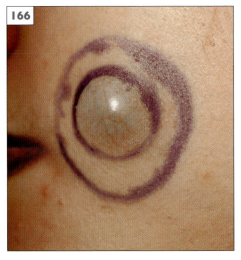

165, 166 Epidermoid cyst.

Epidermoid cysts are common and diagnosis is usually made based on clinical appearance and history. Unusual lesions should be biopsied.

Microscopically, cyst contents are usually made of monomorphic and laminated keratin. Cyst walls typically exhibit thin and cytologically bland epithelial cells. Surrounding irritation (especially lymphocytes) or scarring from previous rupture may be present.

SPECIAL POINTS

Non-inflamed lesions require no treatment, although patients may desire removal for cosmetic reasons. Inflamed lesions should not be directly excised but treated with antibiotics (such a cephalexin or doxycycline), incision and drainage, and culture if necessary. Once the inflammation has settled, excision can be undertaken under local anesthesia. It is important to remove the entire lesion and its exterior sac to decrease the chance of recurrence.

Favre–Racouchot disease

DEFINITION AND CLINICAL FEATURES

Favre–Racouchot disease is a benign, uncommon change to the periocular skin consisting of numerous open comedones ('blackheads') (**168**). It is primarily seen in elderly patients and is believed to be caused by lifetime cumulative sun exposure.

Clinically, numerous, typical open comedones are seen on the temples and periocular cheeks in a setting of chronic sun damage.

EPIDEMIOLOGY

Favre–Racouchot disease is caused by chronic sun exposure. It is more common in males. There may also be an association with smoking.

DIFFERENTIAL DIAGNOSIS AND INVESTIGATIONS

Favre–Racouchot disease is easily distinguished from acne vulgaris since it occurs in adult to elderly patients, consists of only open comedones, and is confined to the periocular skin. The diagnosis is made clinically and further testing is usually not required.

Microscopically, open comedones appear identical to those seen in acne vulgaris. There is usually underlying evidence of sun damage, such as solar elastosis.

SPECIAL POINTS

Treatment with topical retinoids (such as tretinoin cream) is often quite helpful but must be continued indefinitely. Comedone extraction can be helpful, but the lesions often recur. Favre–Racouchot disease is a marker for severe sun damage and patients with this condition should be monitored for skin cancers.

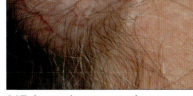

167 Large pilar cyst on scalp.

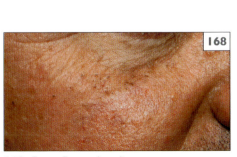

168 Favre–Racouchot disease.

Lipoma

DEFINITION AND CLINICAL FEATURES

Lipomas are common, benign neoplasms of adipose tissue. They can be single or multiple and are generally not clinically significant, although they can be concerning to patients. In some cases, they can also be painful or cosmetically bothersome.

Lipomas generally present as single or multiple, compressible and usually symmetrical deep nodules (**169**). They are often found on the neck, trunk, arms, or thighs. Lesions may grow slowly over time or become irritated with trauma. Angiolipoma, a variant with numerous blood vessels among the fat lobules, is often painful.

EPIDEMIOLOGY

Lipomas are common and frequently incidentally seen in elderly patients.

The cause of lipomas is unknown. There is no known environmental or infectious cause of these lesions. Rarely, multiple lesions can be associated with genetic syndromes such as familial lipoma syndrome or adiposis dolorosa (also called Dercum disease).

DIFFERENTIAL DIAGNOSIS AND INVESTIGATIONS

Lipomas should be differentiated from other subcutaneous tumors. They can mimic benign neoplasms such as epidermal inclusion cysts. They also can be confused with malignant neoplasms such as liposarcoma or metastatic nodules.

The diagnosis is usually made clinically. Lipomas generally feel deeper and less defined than more superficial lesions such as cysts. The overlying skin is usually normal. The lesion will often move easily under the skin such that if pressure is applied over one edge the underlying lipoma will 'slip' away from the pressure. Large or unusual lesions should be excised for histological examination.

Lipomas microscopically consist of normal-appearing adipose cells, which may or may not be surrounded by a thin capsule. Angiolipomas will also feature an above-average number of small and benign-appearing blood vessels.

SPECIAL POINTS

Typical lipomas do not require treatment. Excision can often be easily accomplished either for irritation/discomfort, cosmetic reasons, or to confirm the diagnosis. Traditional excision is effective but can often leave large scars. An alternative technique involves opening a small incision over the lipoma (with a scalpel or punch biopsy) and freeing it from the surrounding tissue, then extracting it from the smaller hole. Liposuction and mesotherapy have also been utilized.

Syringoma

DEFINITION AND CLINICAL FEATURES

Syringomas are common, benign neoplasms of eccrine ducts often found near the eyes. They are of cosmetic concern only.

Syringomas are characterized by multiple, 1–2 mm, flat-topped, flesh-colored papules on the eyelids and periorbital skin (**170**). They can less commonly be found on the trunk and genitals. A rare eruptive presentation with hundreds of lesions has been described.

EPIDEMIOLOGY

Syringomas are more common in females. They may begin at puberty but can occur at any age. The cause of syringomas is not known.

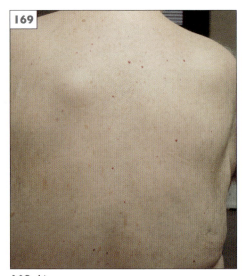

169 Lipoma.

DIFFERENTIAL DIAGNOSIS AND INVESTIGATIONS

Small examples of periocular skin tags, seborrheic keratoses, xanthelasma, and lesions of sebaceous hyperplasia can all be confused with syringomas.

Diagnosis is usually made clinically. Very large or unusual lesions can be biopsied to exclude rare but potentially dangerous adnexal cancers.

Microscopically, syringomas display numerous and benign-appearing small eccrine ducts with amorphous, eosinophilic debris in the lumen.

SPECIAL POINTS

Treatment is not necessary in most cases. Removal for cosmetic reasons is sometimes unsatisfactory, although vaporization with CO_2 laser, electrocautery, and the application of trichloroacetic acid can all be helpful. Recurrence is common.

Dermatofibroma

DEFINITION AND CLINICAL FEATURES

A dermatofibroma is a common, benign neoplasm found on the extremities and sometimes the trunk.

Dermatofibromas appear as solitary to few, 3–10 mm, firm papules, most commonly on the legs but also found on the arms or trunk (**171** & **172**). Lesions may be hyperpigmented, erythematous, or flesh colored.

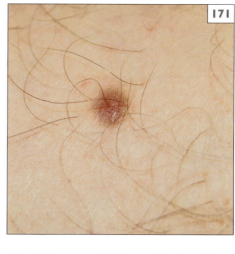

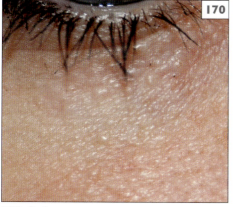

170 Syringoma.

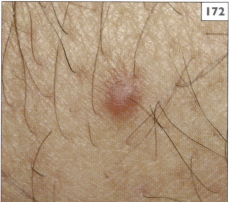

171, 172 Dermatofibroma.

They characteristically exhibit the 'dimple sign' as the epidermis dimples down when squeezed from the lateral edges (**173 & 174**). Most lesions are asymptomatic, but some become irritated or painful. Dermatofibromas on the legs of females may be repeatedly injured by shaving or other hair removal techniques.

EPIDEMIOLOGY

Dermatofibromas are significantly more common in females. Although they develop in younger adulthood, dermatofibromas are persistent unless surgically removed and they tend to be common in elderly patients.

While the exact cause of dermatofibromas is unknown, they may be a form of scar or other benign neoplasm that occurs after minor injuries (such as insect bites or minor trauma). There is no known specific environmental or infectious cause of these lesions.

DIFFERENTIAL DIAGNOSIS AND INVESTIGATIONS

The firm character of dermatofibromas some-times leads to confusion with malignant neoplasms, especially squamous cell carcinoma or skin metastases. Hyperpigmented examples may mimic melanocytic lesions, even melanoma. The malignant version of a dermatofibroma, called dermatofibroma sarcoma protuberans, is usually much larger, deeper, and less defined. Typical scars or small keloid scars can also mimic dermatofibromas. Inflammatory conditions that create firm papules, especially prurigo nodularis and sarcoidosis, can also appear similar.

Diagnosis is generally made clinically based on the location, appearance, and 'dimple sign.' Unusual or large lesions should be biopsied to exclude dermatofibroma sarcoma protuberans or other malignancy.

Microscopically, fascicles of benign-appearing spindle-shaped cells occur in the mid-dermis. There are sometimes associated entrapped collagen fibers.

SPECIAL POINTS

Dermatofibromas are completely benign and generally do not require treatment. Irritated or painful lesions can be treated by surgical removal (often with a punch biopsy under local anesthesia) or cryotherapy.

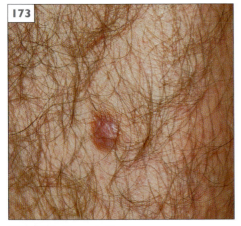
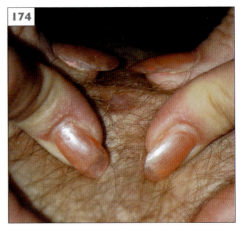

173, 174 Dermatofibroma.

Lentigo

DEFINITION AND CLINICAL FEATURES

A lentigo (plural, lentigines) is a common, benign, melanocytic lesion found on elderly patients. Several forms exist, including simple lentigo (non-sun induced), solar lentigo (sun- or UV radiation induced) (**175**), and mucosal lentigo (**176**). Although common and usually recognizable, these pigmented lesions can cause confusion with more dangerous melanocytic lesions. Lentigines are commonly known to patients as 'liver spots' or 'age spots,' and can be of significant cosmetic concern.

Lentigines present as 3–12 mm, tan to brown, well-demarcated macules. Simple lentigines can occur anywhere on the body. Solar lentigines occur mostly on sun-exposed skin, especially the face, forearms, and dorsal hands. Mucosal lentigines are sometimes more darkly pigmented and occur on the mucosal lips, oral mucosa, penis, and vaginal mucosa.

EPIDEMIOLOGY

All types of lentigines are common and frequently seen in elderly patients.

Simple lentigo is the most common form and is idiopathic. There is no known environmental or infectious cause of simple lentigines. Solar lentigines are induced by UV radiation (either natural sunlight or artificial radiation such as phototherapy or tanning beds) and appear on sun-exposed skin.

Peutz–Jeghers syndrome commonly features multiple oral mucosal lentigines. It is frequently associated with bowel cancer and should be considered in a patient with multiple mucosal lentigines.

DIFFERENTIAL DIAGNOSIS AND INVESTIGATIONS

The main concern with lentigines is differentiating them from melanoma, especially lentigo maligna melanoma, which is especially common on the face in elderly patients, so the distinction is especially important in this population. Macular or thin seborrheic keratoses may also mimic lentigines.

Lentigines are common and usually diagnosed clinically. Large, irregular, or otherwise unusual lesions require biopsy to rule out melanoma. Biopsy of large lesions (which may represent lentigo maligna melanoma in elderly patients) can be difficult to accomplish without disfigurement since these lesions are often on the face.

Microscopically, lentigines exhibit benign-appearing melanocytes with increased pigment visible in those melanocytes and the nearby epidermis.

SPECIAL POINTS

Lentigines are benign and do not require treatment. For lesions of cosmetic concern, cryotherapy is often employed. Several lasers, including Nd:YAG and alexandrite, have been used successfully.

For large lesions that require biopsy, several techniques have been employed. Excisional biopsy is the best choice when possible, since the entire lesion is removed for histological examination. Unfortunately, for large lesions (especially on the face, where lentigo maligna melanoma occurs most frequently) it is often not possible. Incisional biopsy or a series of punch biopsies of the darkest or most irregular areas is sometimes employed. Although these techniques are more cosmetically acceptable, it should be noted that they may sample only more benign-appearing portions of the lesion, potentially leading to a missed diagnosis of melanoma.

175, 176
Lentigo.

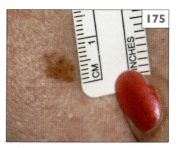

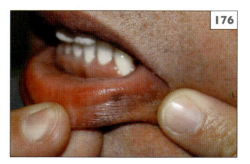

Nevus

DEFINITION AND CLINICAL FEATURES

Nevi are extremely common benign neoplasms of melanocytes found throughout the skin. Nevi are almost ubiquitous and differentiating them from melanoma is a critical aspect of the skin examination. Large or prominent lesions, especially on the face, can be cosmetically concerning to patients. Nevi can also become irritated, especially by chronic friction from body folds, jewelry, or clothing. Dysplastic nevi, which are atypical clinically and/or microscopically but do not meet the criteria for melanoma, are also common.

Nevi present flesh-colored, brown, or black macules or papules anywhere on the skin (**177**). More typical nevi tend to be symmetrical in color and shape, regularly bordered, and less than 6 mm in size. Junctional nevi tend to be macular and more pigmented (**178**), while intradermal nevi tend to be papular and are sometimes flesh colored (**179**).

Features such as asymmetry, jagged or scalloped borders, multiple colors in one lesion, and size greater than 6 mm in diameter are concerning for a dysplastic nevus (**180 & 181**), or even melanoma. The so-called ABCD criteria can be used by both physicians and patients to monitor and evaluate nevi. Some patients have numerous dysplastic nevi, a potential risk factor for melanoma.

There are several subtypes of unusual but benign nevi that may be seen in elderly patients:

- Nevus spilus – a large, regularly brown macule (or café-au-lait macule) with several to dozens of individual 1–2 mm darker-brown junctional nevi (**182**). These lesions should be monitored for growth or changes, but are not frequently precancerous.
- Halo nevus – a typical nevus surrounded by a circular white halo (**183**). Halo nevi occur when the immune system attacks the nevomelanoctyes in the skin, destroying the local pigment (hence the halo) and, eventually, the nevus. Halo nevi are generally not dangerous, but, as with any nevus, should be biopsied if any unusual features are present. Halo nevi in the elderly, which may represent an immune response to melanoma, are vastly more concerning than are nevi in children and adolescents.
- Congenital nevus – a congenital nevus that has been present from birth or shortly thereafter. These nevi can be quite large and often feature course, dark hair growth (**184**). Any large congenital nevi should be closely monitored by the patient and physician for changes. Serial photography is often helpful. Growing or changing lesions should be excised. Larger lesions may require consultation with a plastic surgeon for the best closure options.

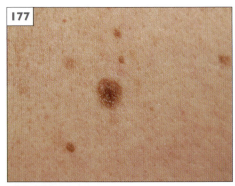

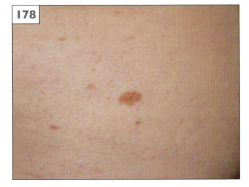

177–178 Nevus.

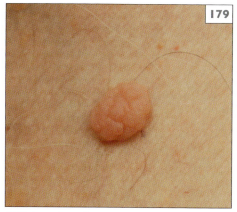

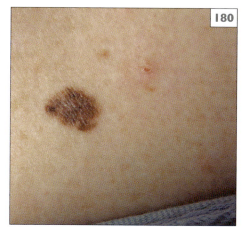

179 Intradermal nevus.

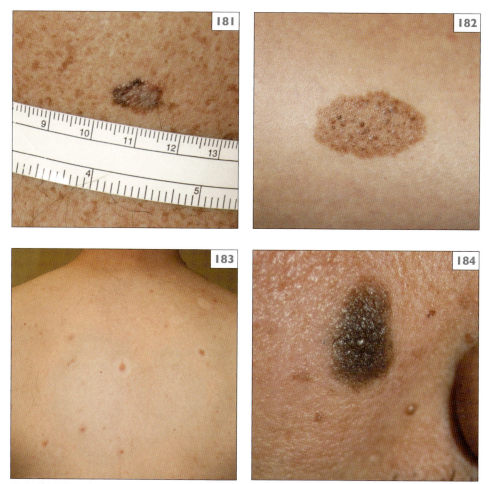

180–184 Dysplastic nevus (**180**); mildly dysplastic nevus (**181**); nevus spilus (**182**); halo nevi (**183**); congenital nevi (**184**).

- Blue nevus – blue nevi are usually small dermal papules with a distinct dark-blue color found often on the scalp or extremities (**185**). If small and typical, they generally do not require treatment. Unusual or large examples should be excised to rule out the rare malignant blue nevus, a form of melanoma.

EPIDEMIOLOGY

Nevi can occur in males and females at any age but often increase in number during young adulthood. They may actually become less common in the very elderly. The exact cause of nevi is unknown, but there is no known infectious or environmental cause. Large numbers of nevi are often seen in hereditary patterns in families. Chronic UV exposure (either sunlight or artificial UV radiation) can lead to an increased number of dysplastic nevi.

DIFFERENTIAL DIAGNOSIS AND INVESTIGATIONS

The key differential diagnosis to consider is melanoma. Although melanoma often meets at least one of the ABCD criteria noted above, it can be subtle in some cases, especially small or amelanotic (non-pigmented) cancers. Other darkly pigmented benign lesions, such as angiomas or angiokeratomas, can simulate junctional nevi. Other flesh-colored papules, such as neurofibromas, fibrous papules, and sebaceous hyperplasia, can mimic intradermal nevi.

Nevi are very common and usually diagnosed clinically. Biopsy of nevi, however, is very commonly used as it can sometimes be difficult to tell benign nevi, dysplastic nevi, and melanoma apart on clinical examination. Dermoscopy can be helpful (if the practitioner is trained in its use) to look for subtle abnormalities that warrant biopsy. Certainly any suspicious or unusual examples should be sampled.

Microscopically, nevi exhibit nests of typical-appearing melanocytes in the epidermis (junctional nevi), dermis (intradermal nevi), or both (compound nevi). Dysplastic examples will have varying levels of cellular and architectural abnormalities, such as single melanocytes, architectural asymmetry, large melanocytes, or large/atypical nuclei.

SPECIAL POINTS

Nevi generally do not require treatment. Cosmetically troublesome lesions can be excised, although the resulting scar may be just as noticeable as the nevus. A shave technique is often utilized for intradermal nevi on the face to avoid a divot scar, although this technique can lead to recurrence since some deeper nevus is usually left behind.

The treatment of dysplastic nevi is controversial, especially as some patients have so many of them as to make excision of all lesions impractical. Some pathology laboratories grade dysplastic nevi as mild, moderate, and severe and will recommend excision for some moderate and all severe lesions. Other laboratories do not grade dysplastic nevi but will still recommend a complete excision for particularly unusual examples. Open communication between the practitioner and the pathologist is critical.

Some dermatologists believe that few dysplastic nevi are truly precancerous themselves, but rather a marker for a patient with an overall increased risk of melanoma. Certainly a patient with a history of dysplastic nevi should undergo regular skin screenings with a physician and perform self-examinations for new or changing lesions.

Photography can also be quite helpful in monitoring nevi. Photographs can be placed in the patient's records and compared with the clinical examination at future visits. This method allows the practitioner to identify new or changing nevi easily, especially if the patient has many lesions.

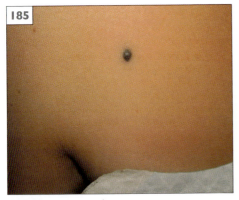

185 Blue nevus on the arm.

Fibrous papule

DEFINITION AND CLINICAL FEATURES

Fibrous papules are common, benign angio-fibromas frequently found on the nose. Although they are completely benign, they can be cosmetically bothersome or mistaken for early skin cancers.

A fibrous papule usually presents as a domed, 1–3 mm, flesh-colored, solitary papule on the face, especially the nasal ala (**186**). They may bleed with minor trauma or scratching. Multiple lesions are less common but sometimes seen.

EPIDEMIOLOGY

Fibrous papules occur commonly in both adult males and females.

The exact cause of fibrous papules is unknown. Some physicians theorize that they are the result of healing from a minor injury. There is no known environmental or infectious cause of fibrous papules.

DIFFERENTIAL DIAGNOSIS AND INVESTIGATIONS

The most common concern with a fibrous papule is to differentiate it from an early non-melanoma skin cancer, especially basal cell carcinoma. Other benign lesions that can mimic a fibrous papule include sebaceous hyperplasia or a small intradermal nevus.

Diagnosis is usually made clinically based on the history (that the lesion is not growing or changing) and the clinical appearance. If there is any suspicion of a skin cancer, a shave biopsy can easily confirm the diagnosis.

Microscopically, fibrous papules exhibit a small papule made of numerous fibroblasts. Fibrosis in the local stroma and dilated blood vessels may also be seen.

SPECIAL POINTS

Fibrous papules are benign and generally do not require treatment. For cosmetically bothersome or suspicious lesions, removal via shave biopsy under local anesthesia is usually satisfactory.

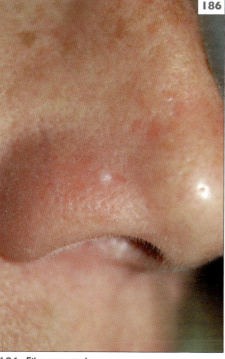

186 Fibrous papule.

Verrucas (warts)

DEFINITION AND CLINICAL FEATURES

Warts are extremely common benign and infectious skin neoplasms caused by human papillomavirus (HPV). Although most common in children, warts are commonly seen in the elderly, especially in immunosuppressed patients. Although not usually dangerous, warts can be cosmetically and functionally bothersome and they can spread both on an individual patient and to others.

Warts are pinpoint to several centimeters in size, verrucous, firm papules, or small plaques. They often rise significantly above the skin and may bleed or hurt with minor trauma. Overlying the wart there are often pinpoint purple or black macules, which represent thrombosed capillaries in the surface of the lesion. Patients often notice these and may refer to them as 'the seeds' of the wart.

There are several common types of warts:

- Common warts – often occur on the face, arms, and hands, but can occur anywhere. They are caused commonly by HPV types 2 and 4 (**187 & 188**).
- Plantar warts – most common on the plantar feet, often deeper and larger than common warts. They are caused commonly by HPV type 1 (**189**).
- Flat warts – small and flat, flesh-colored papules most often seen on the face, dorsal hands, and legs of females who have spread them by shaving. They can be very subtle clinically, even when many lesions are present. They are caused commonly by HPV types 3 and 10.
- Genital warts – sexually transmitted type of HPV-induced wart. They can cause precancerous changes leading to cancer in females (cervical cancer, Bowenoid papulosis) and males (Bowenoid papulosis). They are less common in the elderly, although HPV acquired as a young adult may persist. Pap smears are recommended for all females yearly to monitor for early cervical cancer. They are caused commonly by HPV types 6 and 11 (non-precancerous) and types 16 and 18 (cancerous).

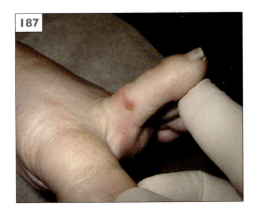

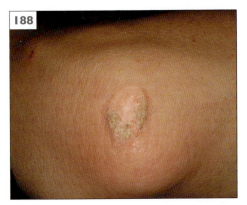

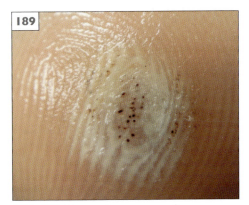

187–189 Verruca (common wart) (**187, 188**); Verruca plantaris (plantar wart) (**189**).

EPIDEMIOLOGY

Warts are extremely common and may occur at any age, although they are most common in children and young adults. Older patients with warts may have a long history of warts (implying an inbred underlying weakness of the patient's immune system against HPV) or history of disease or iatrogenically induced immunosuppression. Warts are commonly seen in transplant recipients for this reason.

DIFFERENTIAL DIAGNOSIS AND INVESTIGATIONS

Warts are often clinically diagnosed, but large, irritated, or unusual variants may be confused with skin cancers, especially squamous cell carcinoma. Warts can also cause a cutaneous horn, which can also arise from an actinic keratosis or squamous cell carcinoma. Seborrheic keratoses are often described as 'warty' and may appear similar, especially smaller examples. Any unusual or suspicious wart should be biopsied for histological confirmation.

Microscopically, warts exhibit papillomatosis, an increased granular layer, dilated capillaries in the upper dermis, and koilocytosis (vacuolated cells). Flat warts can be as subtle microscopically as they are clinically.

SPECIAL POINTS

Warts can be quite difficult to treat and frustrating for both the physician and the patient. Multiple treatments are often required, especially for large or numerous lesions. Commonly employed techniques include liquid nitrogen, cantharidin application, curettage, electrosurgery, bleomycin injection, candida antigen injection, surgical excision, CO_2 or pulsed dye laser, or the application trichloroacetic acid. Several topical treatments are frequently used by the patient at home, including salicylic acid application, imiquimod, fluorouracil, or topical retinoids.

The types of treatment used should be tailored to the location of the warts and the patient's capacity to tolerate any given treatment.

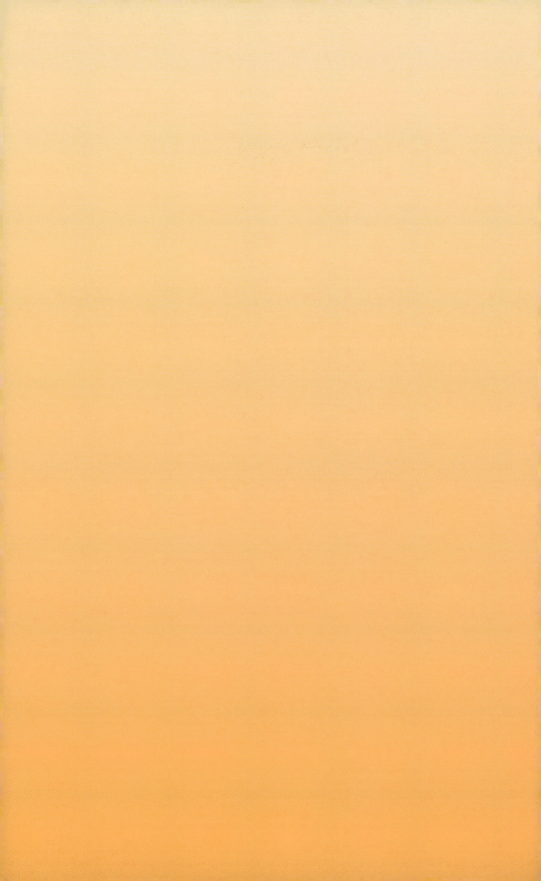

PART 4

Infestations and infections

- **Parasitic**

- **Viral**

- **Bacterial**

- **Fungal**

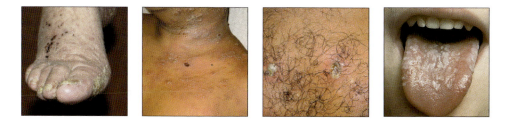

PARASITIC

Scabies

DEFINITION AND CLINICAL FEATURES

Scabies is an infestation caused by a microscopic arthropod, *Sarcoptes scabiei* var. *hominis*. The infestation is caused by the female mite, which can complete her entire life cycle on the skin of a human. After fertilization on the skin surface by a male mite, which dies subsequently, the female burrows into the stratum corneum where she imbibes serum, lays eggs, and defecates. These eggs hatch in 3–5 days. Although about 90% of the hatchlings die, enough will survive to perpetuate the infestation. The female mite, which never again leaves the burrow, herself expires in 1–2 months.

Intense pruritus accompanies scabies infestation. Mite debris and feces are allergenic, and this produces a delayed-type hypersensitivity response. In a primary infestation, several days to a week are required for sensitization before the pruritus begins in earnest, and then it gradually intensifies over weeks. Conversely, in an already sensitized host symptoms may develop in as little as 24–48 hours. Often more than one person in a household may be affected, and this is often an important factor in considering the diagnosis.

The female mite produces small linear burrows no wider than a piece of thread. With a hand lens the female mite can sometimes be visualized as a dot at the end of the burrow. The interdigital areas of the hands and the wrists are involved in 80% of cases of scabies. The interdigital toes and ankles are another common site of involvement (**190 & 191**). Papular lesions may arise in the axillary vault, or on the shaft of the penis, where they are called 'scabetic nodules.' Sometimes these burrows are destroyed by excoriation and a more papulosquamous appearance to the eruption is present (**192 & 193**). The face and neck are spared in most cases of adults.

An otherwise healthy person with scabies has only about a dozen mites on the entire body. Immunocompromised patients (HIV, HTLV), or those unable to scratch (infants and invalids), may have hundreds of thousands of mites, forming plate-like crusts. This variant is called crusted (Norwegian) scabies.

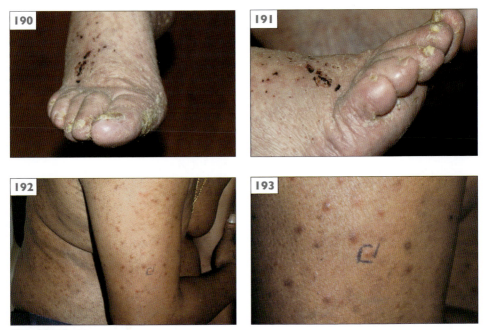

190–193 Scabies.

EPIDEMIOLOGY

Scabies affects about 300 million individuals worldwide. Prevalence rates are higher in developing countries. In the United States, and other developed countries, scabies often occurs in epidemics within nursing homes, hospitals, prisons, and other long-term care facilities.

DIFFERENTIAL DIAGNOSIS AND INVESTIGATIONS

Scabies is just one reason for intense pruritus. Mites that parasitize other animals may occasionally bite a human, but, being unable to complete the entire life cycle on humans, this does not lead to a lasting and perpetual infestation. Prurigo nodularis, a neurodermatitis, is intensely itchy and the scratching and picking lead to marked skin damage. Because some patients with prurigo nodularis also have delusions of parasitosis, this can be a difficult situation to deconstruct. Burrows are not seen in prurigo nodularis.

The diagnosis is confirmed by scraping a burrow lightly with a scalpel blade and then examining the slide under the microscope to visualize the mite, the feces, or the eggs.

SPECIAL POINTS

Scabies is intensely itchy and requires treatment. First-line topical treatments include permethrin cream and lindane. The former is often preferred since lindane has been associated with neurological side effects. The cream is typically applied overnight and washed off in the morning. Treating all members of the household simultaneously and washing/drying linens and clothing worn by the patient may help to prevent re-infestation. Repeating treatment in 5–7 days is also useful since eggs may survive the treatment and hatch subsequently. Since the cream must be applied to the entire body, elderly patients may need assistance with application in difficult to reach areas.

For patients who fail or cannot accomplish topical treatment, oral ivermectin is very effective and usually well tolerated. It is also most effective in treating crusted or Norwegian scabies.

Lice

DEFINITION AND CLINICAL FEATURES

Lice are insects that feed on human blood. Three types of lice infestations include head lice (pediculosis capitis), body lice (pediculosis corporis), and pubic lice (pediculosis pubis). The head louse (*Pediculus humanus capitis*) and the body louse (*P. humanus corporis*) share similar morphologies, while the pubic louse (*Phthirus pubis*) is visually quite distinct. Lice express preference for certain areas of the body based on hair shaft diameter. For this reason, pubic lice may also infest the eyelashes.

- Head lice – most infestations involve one to two dozen adults (3–4 mm) (**194**). The adult female lays eggs (~1 mm), called nits, at the base of the hair shaft. The nits hatch in about a week, and the larvae mature in another 8–9 days. Adult lice are usually located in the postauricular and occipital scalp.
- Body lice – these lice may affect any area of the body, although they tend to avoid the scalp. Usually nits are found in the seams of clothing and not on the body itself, distinguishing it further from a head louse infestation.
- Pubic lice – morphologically resembling crabs (hence the colloquial name), these lice affect the pubic hair and less often the intertriginous hair of adults.

Head lice infestations yield scalp pruritus, occipital lymphadenopathy, and secondary infection. Examination of the scalp often reveals excoriations, nits, and adult lice. A generalized

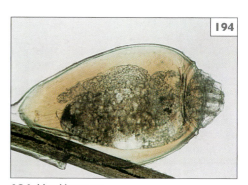

194 Head louse nit.

exanthem has been occasionally described (pityriasis rosea-like pediculid). Body lice and pubic lice often lead to similar findings of pruritus and excoriation. Maculae ceruleae is the name given to hemosiderin-stained, slightly blue, purpuric macules caused by feeding.

EPIDEMIOLOGY

Head lice are found most commonly in school-aged children, typically in late summer and autumn. An estimated 6 million to 12 million infestations occur each year in the United States among children 3–11 years of age. Reported prevalence may be as high as 10–40% in some US schools. White children are more often affected than are black children. Head lice infestations are spread by close person-to-person contact, as the lice crawl and are not capable of jumping or flying. Hair length and personal cleanliness do not impact infestation rates. Animals do not play a role in the transmission of human lice.

Body lice most often occur in people who do not have access to regular bathing and changes of clean clothes, such as the homeless, international refugees, and the victims of war or natural disasters. Body lice can transmit some diseases through biting. Epidemics of typhus and louse-borne relapsing fever have been spread by body lice in areas of social upheaval, and this is an important concern of public health.

Pubic lice are spread through sexual contact and are most common in adults. Pubic lice are sometimes found on the head or eyelashes of pre-pubescent children, and this may be an indication of sexual exposure or abuse. The same consideration would reasonably occur in the geriatric care population.

DIFFERENTIAL DIAGNOSIS AND INVESTIGATIONS

The differential diagnosis of head louse infestations includes monilethrix (a congenital disorder), piedra (an unusual fungal infection forming fungal 'beads' on the hair), and pseudonits (hair casts associated with minor and incidental trauma to the hair). Body louse infestations can be confused with scabies or bed bug bites.

The diagnosis is established by findings of adult lice or nits on the hair or skin, or, in the case of body lice, within the seams of clothing. Lice can crawl rapidly and it may be helpful to fasten a piece of adhesive tape to the infested areas; the lice then stick to the tape and this can be examined under the microscope. Nits fluoresce with a Wood lamp examination and this may assist in the examination of a person with a suspected head louse infestation.

SPECIAL POINTS

Head or pubic lice can be easily treated by shaving the affected area, thereby depriving the lice of their habitat. Body lice will often improve with better routine hygiene, although that may be difficult for very infirm, elderly patients.

Topical treatments include permethrin, pyrethrum, and lindane. Oral ivermectin may be used for cases resistant to topical treatment.

VIRAL

Herpes simplex

DEFINITION AND CLINICAL FEATURES

Herpes simplex virus (HSV) infections are life-long viral infections that present in two general forms:
- Herpes labialis – 'cold sores' or 'fever blisters' around the mouth
- Herpes genitalis – sexually transmitted lesions of the genital region.

Two subtypes of HSV are recognized, namely, HSV-1 and HSV-2. HSV-1 causes >80% of perioral lesions, while HSV-2 causes >80% of genital lesions, but certainly overlap between the subtypes occurs.

During a primary herpes infection, the virus has an incubation period of 2–7 days. Regardless of the location of involvement, lesions of herpes usually appear as small, fluid-filled vesicles on an erythematous base ('dew drops on a rose petal'). Over the next several days lesions may evolve into pustules, crusted papules, or small, punched-out ulcers (**195 & 196**). Finally the lesions heal with minimal scarring.

After resolution of a primary infection, the virus lies dormant within the dorsal root ganglion of the affected dermatome. Subsequent diminutions in immunity, even that of a low-grade fever from a coincidental infection, can cause quiescent herpes to relapse. This led to the colloquial term 'fever blisters' for relapsing herpes labialis. Secondary eruptions occur with varying frequency, depending on the individual and viral subtype, with HSV-2 infections tending to recur more frequently than HSV-1. A prodrome of pain or burning often precedes the relapsing eruption.

EPIDEMIOLOGY

HSV is ubiquitous and infections are seen worldwide. Antibodies to HSV-1 (evidence of exposure but not necessarily clinically apparent disease) correlate with socioeconomic status. By 30 years of age, about 50% of individuals in high socioeconomic circles, but about 80% in lower socioeconomic circles, are seropositive. Antibodies to HSV-2 usually begin to emerge at puberty, and also correlate with sexual activity. Lifetime seroprevalence is about 20–40% of all persons, but is as high as 50–80% of all persons screened at sexually transmitted disease clinics.

DIFFERENTIAL DIAGNOSIS AND INVESTIGATIONS

HSV is usually diagnosed based on clinical appearance and historical information. The differential diagnosis might include ulcerative enanthems, including drug reactions, and bullous impetigo. Chronic perioral herpes infections may be confused with ulcerative squamous cell carcinoma.

Diagnostic modalities include a Tzanck preparation from an intact vesicle, direct fluorescent antibody examination from an intact vesicle, viral culture or PCR analysis, or even histological examination of a skin biopsy.

A Tzanck preparation is obtained by scraping the surface of a freshly unroofed vesicle with subsequent plating and Giemsa staining on a glass microscope slide. If positive, it will demonstrate multinucleated keratinocytes and cytopathic effect, but importantly this does not distinguish between herpes simplex and varicella-zoster infection. In experienced hands, a Tzanck preparation has a sensitivity of around 80%, but the technique is not useful for crusted lesions.

Serum antibodies to HSV are useful for exploring exposure history or for conducting epidemiological surveillance, but they are not typically useful in the acute clinical setting, as titers do not correspond to disease activity.

SPECIAL POINTS

Routine herpes virus infection is usually treated with oral acyclovir (aciclovir), valacyclovir (valaciclovir), or famciclovir. The latter two require less frequent dosing but are more expensive. All three should be used with caution in elderly patients with poor renal function, as they can crystallize in the renal tubules. Topical acyclovir is available for lip lesions.

Widespread or disseminated herpes simplex is very dangerous and often seen in patients with depressed immune systems (including elderly patients). It requires hospitalization and treatment with intravenous acyclovir.

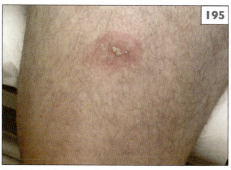
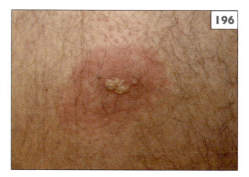

195, 196 Herpes simplex virus.

Varicella-zoster

DEFINITION AND CLINICAL FEATURES

Varicella-zoster virus (VZV) is another viral disease that presents with two different clinical manifestations, depending on whether the infection represents a primary process or recrudescence:

- Primary infection ('chickenpox') – presents in children as a diffuse eruption of pruritic papulovesicles with a truncal predominance.
- Recrudescence ('shingles' or 'zoster') – presents as a painful, vesicular eruption confined to a single dermatome in an elderly and/or immunocompromised patient.

Primary infection with VZV, which is transmitted in respiratory droplets, causes chickenpox. Over 90% of chickenpox occurs before the age of 10 years, so we will not consider it further in this text on skin manifestations within the elderly.

Like herpes simplex virus, VZV lies dormant in the dorsal root ganglion after the manifestations of primary infection have resolved. Years later, as immunity to the virus and overall immune function wanes, the latent virus reactivates, and the proliferating virus travels down axons to the skin. This results in the characteristic painful, vesicular and dermatomal eruption of zoster (**197–200**).

Zoster of the trigeminal nerve is particularly dangerous as it may involve the eye itself. Specifically, involvement of the V1 distribution of the trigeminal nerve, often indicated by involvement of the upper forehead or the tip of the nose (Hutchinson's sign), is an indication for immediate ophthalmic consultation.

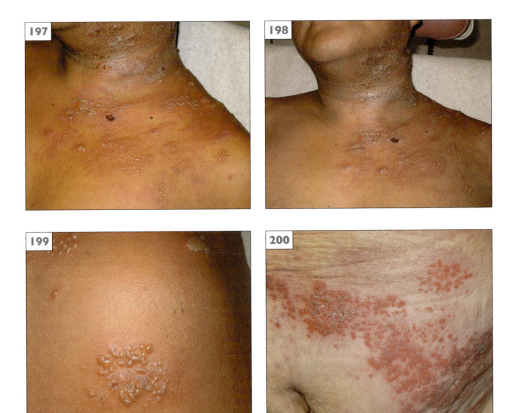

197–200 Varicella-zoster virus.

Recently made available is a live attenuated varicella vaccine that is 14-fold more potent than that of the varicella vaccine used in children. In nearly 40,000 patients >60 years of age enrolled in the vaccine trial, the burden of zoster dropped 61% in comparison with the control group. Furthermore, the incidence of post-herpetic neuralgia dropped 67%. The vaccine offers protection for at least 4 years, but it is unknown whether beyond this it will completely prevent zoster or more simply just delay onset to a later age. Nevertheless, this vaccine is an available option for elderly patients who wish to reduce their risk of developing zoster and possible post-herpetic neuralgia.

EPIDEMIOLOGY

The lifetime risk of zoster is about 10–20%. Recrudescence serves as a 'booster' to the immune system, and therefore, most patients will have only a single episode of zoster in a lifetime. Older patients, particularly those who experience significant pain with the eruption of zoster, can develop post-herpetic neuralgia that persists, by definition, more than 30 days after resolution of the skin lesions.

The incidence of post-herpetic neuralgia in patients with zoster who are >60 years old is about 40%, while the incidence in those <60 years old is about 10%.

DIFFERENTIAL DIAGNOSIS AND INVESTIGATIONS

The pain of zoster often precedes the actual eruption and when this occurs in a thoracic dermatome it has even been confused with myocardial infarction. A Tzanck preparation performed on cells scraped from the base of a freshly unroofed blister may reveal diagnostic epidermal changes including multinucleated keratinocytes and cytopathic effect.

As mentioned previously, these changes are common to both herpes simplex virus and VZV infections. Clinical information and/or viral culture, PCR, or direct fluorescence exam results may be used to discriminate between the two conditions. VZV culture is technically demanding and has a relatively low sensitivity.

SPECIAL POINTS

Typical re-activation varicella (shingles) is usually treated with a course of oral acyclovir (aciclovir) or valacyclovir (valaciclovir). Since the condition is often quite painful, topical lidocaine as a cream or gel may be useful. Narcotics are sometimes required but should be used with caution in elderly patients where they may cause disorientation or falls. Severe or persistent pain (post-herpetic neuralgia) may benefit from consultation with a pain management specialist, since antidepressants, antiseizure medications, and long-term narcotics may be helpful.

Patients with active lesions should avoid contact with pregnant females and unvaccinated children since they may spread the virus (and cause chickenpox) in non-immune persons.

A vaccine for recurrent VZV is available and recommended for patients over 60 years of age to prevent shingles.

Disseminated VZV is very dangerous and often seen in patients with depressed immune systems (including elderly patients). It requires hospitalization and treatment with intravenous acyclovir. Primary VZV can also be quite dangerous (especially due to pneumonitis) in the elderly, although it is unusual for an elderly person not to already be immune from previous exposure.

BACTERIAL

Bacterial cellulitis/Erysipelas

DEFINITION AND CLINICAL FEATURES

Bacterial cellulitis is an acute infection of the skin and soft tissue characterized by localized edema, erythema, warmth, and pain (**201**). Often this erythema expands as the cellulitis progresses to involve more tissue. The condition usually follows a break in the skin, such as a fissure, cut, laceration, or insect bite.

Most cases of cellulitis are caused by *Staphylococcus aureus* or *Streptococcus pyogenes*. Cases caused by *Streptococcus pyogenes* often present with brighter erythema, sharper demarcation, brawny edema, and are referred to as erysipelas (**202**). Erysipelas often involves the face or lower extremities. Regional lymphadenopathy is common with erysipelas, and systemic symptoms including malaise, fever, and chills may occur.

EPIDEMIOLOGY

Cellulitis is a common infection seen worldwide. Obesity, diabetes, and poor lymphatic drainage predispose to cellulitis. Tinea pedis, when coupled with one of the aforementioned conditions, may render one even more vulnerable to recurrent episodes of cellulitis, likely due to chronic fissuring in the feet.

Mortality rate with most forms of cellulitis is low (<5%), but death may occur in neglected cases or when the infection is caused by highly virulent organisms, like *Pseudomonas aeruginosa*. Factors associated with an increased risk of death include congestive heart failure, morbid obesity, hypoalbuminemia, or concurrent illness.

DIFFERENTIAL DIAGNOSIS AND INVESTIGATIONS

The diagnosis of cellulitis is based primarily on the clinical presentation. It is not unusual to 'ink and date' (place marks with a pen on the skin) the margins of the erythema to monitor for extension or improvement. While once touted, aspiration and culture at the edge of the erythematous area yield a positive result in only about 30% of the cases; a negative study does not exclude the possibility of cellulitis.

A CBC may be useful as an adjunctive test in questionable cases. Typically laboratory investigations reveal a leukocytosis (>10,000 cells/mm^3) and fever in about one-half of cases. Blood cultures should be routinely performed to exclude septicemia, which occurs in up to 2–10% of cases. The utility of a biopsy is limited as bacteria are infrequently identified and the histology is often non-specific.

Among the other diagnostic considerations is necrotizing fasciitis, a more dangerous and often fatal condition caused by many different bacteria. This more deeply situated infection progresses rapidly and often presents with pain out of proportion to that of typical cellulitis. Bilateral involvement militates somewhat against infection, and favors other causes of edema and erythema, such as venous stasis dermatitis.

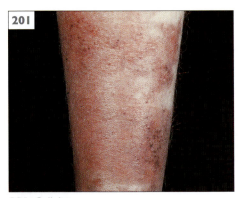

201 Cellulitis.

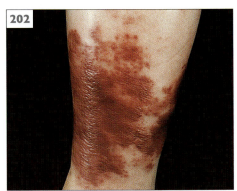

202 Erysipelas.

SPECIAL POINTS

Systemic antibiotics are the mainstay of treatment for bacterial skin infections. Given the high level of penicillin resistance in bacteria today, first-line treatment is often with a cephalosporin (such as cephalexin), TMP/SMX, or tetracycline derivative.

Elderly patients may be particularly prone to sepsis arising from cellulitis. Severe infections or those complicated by chronic illness, diabetes, or vascular insufficiency should be considered for hospitalization and intravenous antibiotics.

Bacterial folliculitis

DEFINITION AND CLINICAL FEATURES

Bacterial folliculitis is an infection of the follicular unit. Depending on the depth of the process, a variety of clinical manifestations may result:

- Superficial folliculitis – small, erythematous papules and fragile pustules located on the trunk, extremities, scalp, or face (**203 & 204**).
- Furuncle/furunculosis – more substantial infection of the hair follicle that also involves the surrounding subcutis (**205**).
- Carbuncle/carbunculosis – coalescence of furuncles producing a subcutaneous abscess, which may be associated with systemic symptoms.

Most folliculitis is caused by *Staphylococcus aureus*. Gram-negative bacteria may cause some isolated cases of folliculitis, particularly in the anogenital region or in patients placed on chronic tetracycline-based therapy for acne. Painful and rapidly evolving lesions may also be suspicious for CA-MRSA.

Up to around a quarter of patients with bacterial folliculitis may experience recurrent disease, and the rise of CA-MRSA also contributes to this phenomenon.

Recreational folliculitis ('hot-tub folliculitis') is caused by transient infection with *Pseudomonas aeruginosa* from poorly chlorinated hot tubs or swimming pools, and in the elderly, this might also encompass disease spread through heated therapeutic whirlpools as well.

EPIDEMIOLOGY

Folliculitis is quite common, but, because the superficial forms of the disease are often self-limited or considered inconsequential, many cases do not present to the doctor. Certain conditions

or behaviors may make patients more susceptible to folliculitis including frequent shaving, immuno-suppression, pre-existing dermatoses, long-term antibiotic use, occlusive clothing and/or occlusive dressings, exposure to hot humid temperatures, diabetes mellitus, and obesity.

DIFFERENTIAL DIAGNOSIS AND INVESTIGATIONS

Typically the diagnosis of bacterial folliculitis is based on the clinical presentation and historical information. Both deep-seated fungal infections

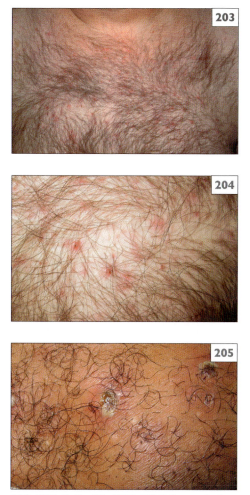

203–205 Folliculitis (**203, 204**); furunculosis (**205**).

and herpetic viral folliculitis must be considered in the differential. In an era of increasing bacterial resistance, culture of the contents of pustules may confirm the diagnosis and also provide valuable information on antibiotic susceptibility. This is particularly true for cases that are more severe, for cases that have not responded adequately to treatment, or for cases involving the anogenital area, where Gram-negative infection is more common. The increasing prevalence of CA-MRSA has also highlighted the importance of obtaining a culture.

SPECIAL POINTS

Mild folliculitis is common and does not necessarily require treatment. Antibacterial soaps used for bathing may be helpful in treating mild cases and preventing recurrence.

For mild cases, topical antibiotics (such as clindamycin lotion or solution) may be helpful. For more severe outbreaks, systemic antibiotics are usually required. A swab culture of a few typical lesions may be helpful in targeting antibiotic treatment, especially if *S. aureus* is the cause. For recurrent cases, long-term antibiotics may be required.

For the most severe cases systemic isotretinoin may be useful, although it is not always well tolerated in elderly patients.

FUNGAL

Tinea

DEFINITION AND CLINICAL FEATURES

Tinea infections are caused by superficial fungi called dermatophytes that are capable of using keratin within the sloughed skin of the stratum corneum as an energy substrate. These infections may be acquired from other humans (anthropophilic), from animals (zoophilic), or from the soil (geophilic).

Tinea is often referred to by laypersons as 'ringworm' as it produces intensely pruritic, annular lesions with peripheral scale, central clearing, and variable inflammation. Tinea is often subclassified based on the body region involved, and the most common forms in general dermatology include:
- Tinea corporis – dermatophyte infection of the body, often forms annular scaling plaques with central clearing and surrounding erythema. The lesions may be small and numerous (**206**) or large and ill defined (**207**).
- Tinea capitis – dermatophyte infection of the scalp, often results in alopecia and occipital lymphadenopathy. If the inflammation is substantial, a kerion (scarring) will result in permanent hair loss. Tinea capitis is unusual in adults.
- Tinea pedis – dermatophyte infection of the feet. It can present as either a moist and macerated interdigital form (**208**), or in the elderly in particular it may yield a dry, hyperkeratotic and minimally erythematous eruption on the entire surface of the foot ('moccasin-like tinea pedis') (**209**).
- Tinea cruris – dermatophyte infection of the groin, seen almost exclusively in males. The annular eruption tends to spread on the highly keratinized skin of the medial thigh and spares the light-keratinized scrotum in a pattern opposite to that of cutaneous candidiasis (**210**).

EPIDEMIOLOGY

Tinea infections are common worldwide. In fact, tinea pedis is the most common fungal infection of mankind. Chronic moisture may predispose to tinea, and, hence, tinea infections are often more pervasive and extensive in humid and tropical regions. Diabetics are particularly prone to tinea infections, as are patients using immunosuppressive medications, including high-dose prednisone.

Prior misdiagnosis, and mistaken treatment with topical steroids, may alter the clinical appearance of tinea. While topical steroids initially lessen the inflammation and decrease

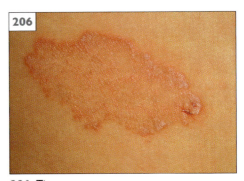

206 Tinea.

pruritus, they suppress the local immune response, thereby perpetuating the infection.

DIFFERENTIAL DIAGNOSIS AND INVESTIGATIONS

Tinea is often suspected based on the clinical presentation of an intensely pruritic, annular, and scaling eruption. A history of exposure to new pets or environments associated with tinea infections (health clubs, hotels, and so on) may be helpful in suggesting the source of the infection.

A KOH preparation of scale taken from the edge of an annular lesion should reveal hyphal elements when examined under the microscope. For tinea capitis, material for a KOH preparation may be obtained by vigorously rubbing the area with a moistened piece of gauze, swab, or even sterile toothbrush. Fungal culture of scrapings is also useful, but the results take several days to weeks to obtain.

SPECIAL POINTS

Minor superficial fungal infections are common in elderly patients and do not require treatment if not bothersome. Topical antifungals (such as miconazole or clotrimazole cream) are numerous and often quite useful. The patient can keep them handy since these infections are often recurrent.

More severe or widespread tinea skin infections can be treated with a short course of oral antifungals (terbinafine or itraconazole). These medications can be harmful to the liver and should be avoided in patients with underlying liver disease or heavy alcohol use. Itraconazole also has numerous drug interactions and may be difficult to use in elderly patients already on many other medications.

Fungal nail infections require longer-term treatment with oral medications (typically 6 weeks for fingernails and 3 months for toenail infections). Recurrence is common. Topical treatment of onychomycosis is usually unsatisfactory owing to poor penetration of the thick nail. For painful or disfigured nails, filing, clipping, and consultation with a podiatrist may be helpful.

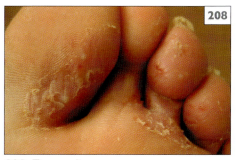

208 Tinea pedis.

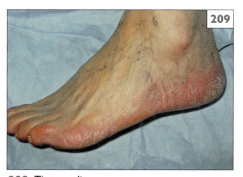

209 Tinea pedis.

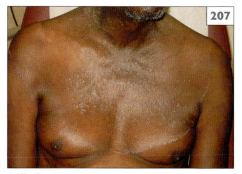

207 Tinea corporis.

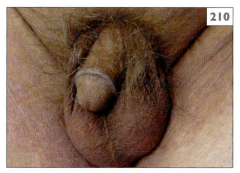

210 Tinea cruris.

Candidiasis

DEFINITION AND CLINICAL FEATURES

Cutaneous candidiasis is a superficial skin infection caused chiefly by the yeast, *Candida albicans*, although rare forms of *Candida* species might be involved in occasional cases. *Candida* is a normal commensal organism of many skin surfaces, but in pathological circumstances it becomes vastly overgrown.

Similar to tinea infections, different names are assigned to cutaneous candidiasis, depending on the site of infection. Candida infection involving the axilla, or inguinal or inframammary folds is called candidal intertrigo (**211**), but this is distinct from simple intertrigo, which is an irritant process. Disease involving the oral mucosa is referred to as thrush (**212**) and candida infection involving the oral commisure is called perleche.

In all forms of cutaneous infection, *Candida* tends to induce the formation of 'beef-red,' highly inflammatory plaques, often with surrounding satellite pustules. Pruritus is a common complaint.

EPIDEMIOLOGY

Tinea occurs all over the world, and is particularly prevalent in humid tropical environments. Moisture predisposes to candidiasis, and this is one reason that the intertriginous sites of the body are so often involved. It also means that tinea is more common in the groin area of elderly patients with incontinence. Patients with diabetes or people on chronic antibiotic regimens may also be predisposed to candida infection, likely due to hyperglycemia and a lack of competition from normal skin bacteria, respectively.

DIFFERENTIAL DIAGNOSIS AND INVESTIGATIONS

Simple intertrigo is caused by the irritant effect of sweat in the bodily folds, but does not have a component of candida overgrowth. Tinea cruris can be confused with candidiasis but tends to spare the scrotum and lacks the same brightly erythematous and pustular response. A KOH skin preparation is confirmatory, simple and cost-effective, which allows visualization of yeast and pseudohyphae.

SPECIAL POINTS

Thorough drying of affected areas after bathing and use of drying agents (such as skin powders) is often helpful. Minor candida skin infections can usually be treated topically (clotrimazole cream is especially active against *Candida*).

More severe infections can be treated systemically with fluconazole. As with other azole antifungal medications, it has many potential drug interactions, which are especially likely in elderly patients who may be on many medications and have diminished liver function.

Disseminated candida infection is very dangerous and typically requires hospital admission and treatment with intravenous antifungals (such as amphotericin or voriconazole).

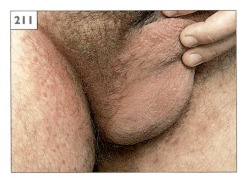

211 Candidal intertrigo.

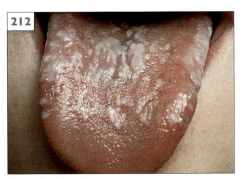

212 Oral thrush.

PART 5

Metabolic and nutritional disease

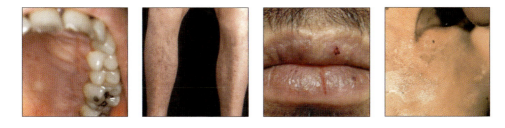

Scurvy

DEFINITION AND CLINICAL FEATURES

Scurvy is chronic deficiency of vitamin C (ascorbic acid), which typically causes bleeding in the gums (**213**), skin, joints, and muscles due to improper collagen formation. Although rare, scurvy is important to recognize in the elderly both because it is easily treatable and because it may be a sign of other significant problems, such as alcoholism or neglect.

Skin signs of scurvy include petechiae (including perifollicular petechiae), bruising, and the formation of 'corkscrew hairs' (**214**). Other common findings include anemia and swollen, friable gums that bleed easily.

EPIDEMIOLOGY

Scurvy is rare in the Western world, as many foods are fortified with vitamin C and citrus fruit is widely available.

Scurvy occurs several months after vitamin C is withdrawn from the diet. It primarily occurs in children being fed strict diets, the elderly, alcoholics, and others whose nutrition is compromised. Elderly patients are frequent targets of scurvy as they have several potential reasons to limit their diets, including loss of teeth, difficulty swallowing or chewing, living alone without access to fresh foods, or comorbidities such as alcoholism or dementia.

DIFFERENTIAL DIAGNOSIS AND INVESTIGATIONS

The differential diagnosis of scurvy includes other conditions that cause easy bleeding, including medication (aspirin, warfarin), thrombocytopenia, and leukemia. As noted previously, the skin of the elderly may also be prone to easy bruising without specific pathology due to age-related fat loss and skin thinning.

Although scurvy can be suspected clinically, confirmation requires a blood test for ascorbic acid levels. A CBC and other vitamin levels (especially vitamin B_{12} and folate) are advisable for patients with scurvy.

SPECIAL POINTS

Scurvy can lead to fatal hemorrhage if untreated, so suspected cases should be tested and treated immediately. Following vitamin C supplementation, symptoms of scurvy usually resolve within a few days.

In elderly patients, it is critical to understand why scurvy occurred. If the patient is suffering from neglect, dementia, alcoholism, or any other condition leading to malnutrition, then that condition needs to be dealt with to avoid recurrence.

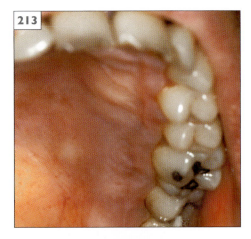

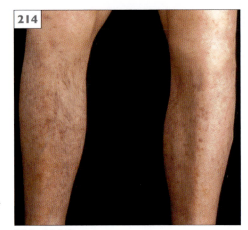

213, 214 Scurvy.

Cheilitis

DEFINITION AND CLINICAL FEATURES
Cheilitis is inflammation of the lip and has many potential causes. Angular cheilitis refers to inflammation only at the corners of the mouth. Several of the potential causes of cheilitis are more common in the elderly.

Clinically, cheilitis is present when the common signs of inflammation are present on the lips and nearby skin, including erythema, pain, or tenderness, cracking, or scaling (**215**). It is important to perform a complete history and physical examination to look for potential causes.

EPIDEMIOLOGY
Cheilitis is a common complaint in the elderly. Potential causes that are more common in elderly patients include chronic sun exposure (actinic cheilitis), malnutrition (riboflavin, iron, or vitamin B_{12} deficiency), and candida overgrowth.

DIFFERENTIAL DIAGNOSIS AND INVESTIGATIONS
The differential diagnosis of cheilitis is extensive.

Actinic cheilitis is caused by chronic sun exposure and analogous to actinic keratoses on the skin. It is important that this precancerous change be treated, since resulting squamous cell carcinoma of the lip is at high risk for metastasis. Biopsy is warranted if there is any suspicion of squamous cell carcinoma.

Malnutrition is also a potential cause of cheilitis in the elderly. Patients with underlying medical problems such as swallowing difficulties, dental problems, neglect, dementia, or alcoholism may not eat a varied diet and may become deficient in riboflavin, vitamin B_{12}, zinc, or iron. If these causes are suspected, blood testing of the relevant vitamin levels and supplementation should be undertaken. It is also important to treat the underlying cause, when possible, to prevent recurrence.

Allergic contact dermatitis to chemicals in lipstick, facial products, flavorings, or metallic dental appliances may cause cheilitis. Patch testing may be performed to exclude these causes.

Perlèche, an overgrowth of *Candida albicans*, is a common cause of angular cheilitis. It can usually be controlled with antiyeast therapy, such as topical clotrimazole cream or clotrimazole troches.

Medications can also cause cheilitis, especially chemotherapy agents and systemic retinoids (such as acitretin for psoriasis or bexarotene for lymphoma).

SPECIAL POINTS
The treatment of cheilitis requires a careful search for its underlying cause. Emollient lip products, such as plain petrolatum or a mild steroid ointment, may also be helpful. Sunscreen applied to the lips should be encouraged for patients when outdoors.

It is important to exclude (by examination or biopsy) actinic cheilitis, which is a precancerous form of sun damage and requires treatment. Actinic cheilitis is most often treated with liquid nitrogen, fluorouracil cream, or imiquimod cream.

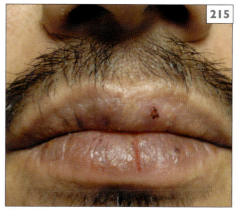

215 Cheilitis.

Pruritus

DEFINITION AND CLINICAL FEATURES

Pruritus (itching) is a frequent complaint among elderly patients. It can present from mild to very severe, with the latter often being very debilitating. Pruritus has many causes, and workup and treatment should be guided by the history and physical examination. A complete history, including the location, duration, and severity of the itching, will be helpful in targeting the examination.

Itching may be present without any clinical features or with only primary excoriations. It is important to check for subtle signs of skin problems, such as xerosis (skin dryness), scabies, or a drug eruption, as the itching will persist until the underlying condition is treated.

EPIDEMIOLOGY

Itching is very common in patients of all ages but especially common in the elderly. It occurs in both males and females.

DIFFERENTIAL DIAGNOSIS AND INVESTIGATIONS

The differential diagnosis of pruritus is extensive. A thorough history and physical examination should guide attempts at testing and treatment. Common causes in the elderly include dry skin, drug reactions, scabies, metabolic imbalance, internal malignancy, and psychogenic causes.

First, an attempt to diagnose any underlying dermatosis should be made. Any visible skin eruption should be examined and potentially biopsied. Empiric treatment for conditions like scabies may be warranted, as diagnosis may sometimes be difficult even with a complete examination and biopsy. When an underlying dermatosis has been excluded, laboratory testing may be helpful (*Table 2*).

Examination by a primary care physician with age-appropriate cancer screening is warranted if other causes of itching are excluded.

SPECIAL POINTS

The treatment of pruritus in the elderly begins with attempting to diagnose its cause. If a diagnosis can be made then treatment of the underlying condition is the first course of action.

In cases where no diagnosis is found despite exhaustive search or when the diagnosis is not treatable, symptomatic treatment of itching can make an enormous difference in the patient's quality of life.

Initial treatments include gentle skin care and emollients. Patients should be advised to bathe as little as possible in warm but not hot water. Harsh, drying, or perfumed soaps should be avoided. Liberal amounts of moisturizer should be applied to the skin daily, ideally something occlusive such as petrolatum. Proper oral hydration should be encouraged.

When these conservative measures are insufficient, medical treatment should be initiated. A non-sedating antihistamine for morning use with a sedating antihistamine (such as hydroxyzine or doxepin) at bedtime is often helpful. Routine antihistamines are usually more useful than ones taken only when itching occurs. Sedating antihistamines should be monitored closely in elderly patients, since they can lead to confusion or falls.

Phototherapy is often useful for itching. Narrow-band UVB is a relatively safe choice in elderly patients with severe itching. Often several weeks of treatment are needed to see benefit and it may need to be continued long term to maintain results.

Table 2
Laboratory testing related to pruritis

Laboratory test	Potential condition causing pruritus
CBC	Anemia, leukemia, polycythemia vera
Thyroid-stimulating hormone	Hypothyroidism, Graves disease
Complete metabolic profile	Hepatic or renal disease, cholestasis
Ferritin	Iron deficiency
Helicobacter pylori antibody	Gastric *H. pylori* infection
HIV antibody	HIV infection
Hepatitis B and C antibodies	Chronic hepatitis
ESR	Underlying systemic inflammation, lupus
ANAs	Underlying connective tissue disease

When itching is severe and persistent, more aggressive medical therapy, such as systemic steroids or naltrexone, can be tried. It is important to balance the potential benefits of such treatments against risks and the patient's comorbidities.

Zinc deficiency

DEFINITION AND CLINICAL FEATURES
Zinc deficiency is rare in the Western world and is caused by insufficient dietary intake or abnormally increased consumption of the mineral. Elderly patients are at increase risk for zinc deficiency due to potential underlying causes of malnutrition.

Zinc deficiency causes brightly erythematous, sharply defined, and scaly plaques around the mouth, perianal skin, and skin flexures (**216 & 217**). There may also be associated alopecia and a red, glossy tongue.

EPIDEMIOLOGY
Although zinc deficiency is rare, the elderly are at increased risk due to problems including swallowing difficulties, dental issues, neglect, dementia, or alcoholism. Zinc deficiency can also occur in the setting of increased zinc consumption due to injury or illness.

DIFFERENTIAL DIAGNOSIS AND INVESTIGATIONS
Zinc deficiency may appear similar to psoriasis (especially inverse psoriasis), candidiasis or tinea, and eczema. Serum zinc levels may be tested if it is suspected.

SPECIAL POINTS
Treatment is with supplemental zinc (either dietary or intravenous) and is usually effective quite quickly. It is important to treat the underlying cause, when possible, to prevent recurrence.

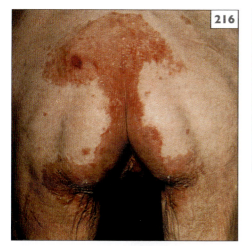
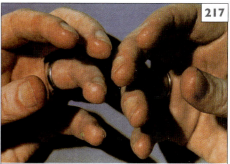

216, 217 Zinc deficiency. Reproduced from: Freedberg, Irwin, *Fitzpatrick's Dermatology in General Medicine*, 5/e © 1998 with permission from the McGraw-Hill Companies.

Pellagra

DEFINITION AND CLINICAL FEATURES

Pellagra is chronic deficiency of the B vitamin niacin. It may occur from either deficiency of niacin or tryptophan in the diet. Tryptophan can be converted to niacin in the body if intake is sufficient.

Pellagra is classically associated with the four Ds: dermatitis, dementia, diarrhea, and death. Itching and scaling occur on the sun-exposed skin and may progress to lichenification and hyperpigmentation (**218**). These changes are often sharply demarcated on the arms and neck (the so-called Casal necklace).

EPIDEMIOLOGY

Pellagra is rare in the Western world where dietary intake of niacin is usually more than sufficient. The elderly, however, are at increased risk due to problems including swallowing difficulties, dental issues, neglect, dementia, and alcoholism.

DIFFERENTIAL DIAGNOSIS AND INVESTIGATIONS

The differential diagnosis of pellagra includes other sharply demarcated or photodistributed dermatoses such as photodrug reactions or photocontact dermatitis.

Low serum levels of niacin or urine levels of its metabolites establish the diagnosis. Patients with typical symptoms should be started on replacement immediately while laboratory studies are pending.

SPECIAL POINTS

Treatment is with supplemental niacin (or niacinamide) and is usually effective quite quickly. It is important to treat the underlying cause, when possible, to prevent recurrence.

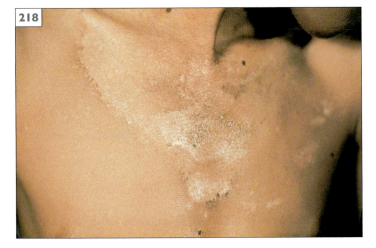

218 Pellagra.

PART 6

Skin signs of systemic disease

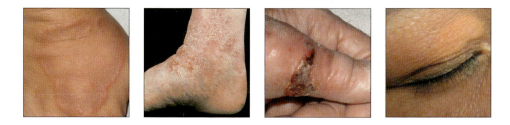

Necrobiosis lipoidica (diabeticorum)

DEFINITION AND CLINICAL FEATURES

Necrobiosis lipoidica is a granulomatous and necrobiotic disorder of collagen that affects the skin of the anterior pretibial surfaces. It is associated with diabetes mellitus. The disease results in a thinned and atrophic epidermis with yellowish, discolored plaques and dilated underlying vessels (**219**). Ulcerations may occur easily with trauma given the atrophic nature of the skin. Usually the lesions are multiple and bilateral. Although sometimes painful, often the patient's chief complaint is the unsightly cosmetic appearance of the lesions.

EPIDEMIOLOGY

Necrobiosis lipoidica occurs in about 0.3% of diabetic patients. In patients with necrobiosis lipoidica, the skin changes precede diabetes in about 15%, follow the diagnosis of diabetes in 60%, and occur concomitantly with the diagnosis of diabetes in about 25%. When associated with diabetes the presence or even the progression of necrobiosis lipoidica does not correlate with glycemic control.

Necrobiosis lipoidica is three times more common in females than males. The average age of onset is 30 years, but it can occur at any age, including later life. The disease tends to develop at an earlier age in patients with diabetes, when compared with cryptogenic cases.

DIFFERENTIAL DIAGNOSIS AND INVESTIGATIONS

The differential diagnosis includes granuloma annulare, profound stasis dermatitis (possibly with lipodermatosclerosis), pretibial myxedema, and erythema nodosum. A punch biopsy is of high utility in discriminating between these diagnostic possibilities. Laboratory findings are not particularly helpful in the diagnosis of necrobiosis lipoidica, although some experts advocate glucose tolerance testing or other screening methods to exclude diabetes mellitus.

SPECIAL POINTS

Necrobiosis lipoidica is poorly understood and can be difficult to treat. Potent topical steroids under occlusion or intralesional steroids are often first-line treatment. Systemic steroids may be helpful, but are often difficult to use in diabetic or elderly patients. Phototherapy may be helpful in resistant cases.

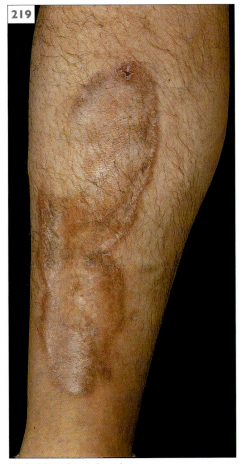

219 Necrobiosis lipoidica.

Acanthosis nigricans

DEFINITION AND CLINICAL FEATURES

Acanthosis nigricans is a cutaneous manifestation of internal disease that occurs in two principle situations:

- Classic – a benign variant associated with obesity and insulin resistance.
- Paraneoplastic – a malignant variant in association with cancer.

Classic acanthosis nigricans presents as hyperpigmented, slightly velvety, thickened skin on the nape of the neck, the axillae, the groin, and other flexural surfaces (**220**). The malignant form of acanthosis nigricans is often more explosive and may involve, in addition to involvement of the classic sites, the mucosal surfaces as well. Malignant acanthosis nigricans may present concomitantly with the sign of Leser–Trélat (explosive onset of multiple seborrheic keratoses).

EPIDEMIOLOGY

Classic acanthosis nigricans, being associated with obesity, continues to increase in the United States, as does obesity. More than one-half of persons weighing more than double their ideal body weight have acanthosis nigricans. The disorder is more common in people with darker skin types. For example, the prevalence in white people is <1%, whereas in Hispanic and black people, the prevalence is 6% and 13%, respectively. Malignant acanthosis is rather rare, but is most often associated with gastrointestinal malignancy.

DIFFERENTIAL DIAGNOSIS AND INVESTIGATIONS

The diagnosis of acanthosis nigricans is usually established clinically. The differential diagnosis includes, among other entities, intertrigo, tinea, and erythrasma. A biopsy is not usually helpful.

Patients with acanthosis nigricans should be screened for diabetes. One superior screening test for insulin resistance is the plasma insulin level, which will be high in those with resistance. This is the most sensitive test because many younger patients will not yet have overt diabetes or an abnormal glycated hemoglobin level, but they will have a high plasma insulin level. For those with symptoms of frank diabetes standard screening labs and a glycated hemoglobin level are appropriate.

To exclude malignant acanthosis nigricans, the first step is a careful history, review of systems, and age-appropriate cancer screening. Other screening tests can be undertaken based on the results of these preliminary maneuvers.

SPECIAL POINTS

Treatment of the skin lesions of acanthosis nigricans is generally not necessary and can be very difficult. It is important to advise the patient on maintaining a healthy weight, exercise, and routine glucose monitoring due to the prevalence of diabetes and glucose intolerance in these patients. Topical acid preparations, such as ammonium lactate lotion, may help smooth the skin.

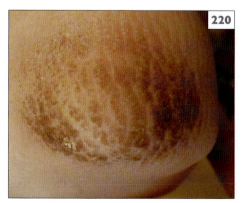

220 Acanthosis nigricans.

Granuloma annulare

DEFINITION AND CLINICAL FEATURES

Granuloma annulare is an inflammatory disorder that typically presents as dermal papules and annular plaques. Most cases are idiopathic and limited, presenting usually on the distal extremities (**221 & 222**). However, some cases of generalized granuloma annulare are associated with systemic disease, particularly diabetes mellitus, and, to a lesser extent, hepatitis C and HIV.

The generalized form of granuloma annulare is most germane to our discussion of skin signs of systemic disease. It presents with a few to innumerable papules (2–8 mm) that range in color from erythematous to flesh-colored. These lesions may coalesce into annular plaques of several centimeters' diameter (**223**). As it is a dermal process, there is no overlying scale or other epidermal changes.

EPIDEMIOLOGY

Generalized granuloma annulare comprises <10% of all cases of the disease, annulare, and it demonstrates a bimodal age distribution. It occurs sometimes in patients <10 years of age (similar to more isolated and 'classic' disease), but more often in patients aged 30–60 years of age.

DIFFERENTIAL DIAGNOSIS AND INVESTIGATIONS

When the papules of generalized granuloma annulare coalesce into annulare plaques, the differential diagnosis might include tinea, although granuloma annulare is not scaly and is not as pruritic as most fungal infections. Laboratory studies are largely non-contributory in patients with granuloma annulare, even in generalized disease, but, given the association with diabetes, screening is often appropriate. Other testing to exclude hepatitis C and HIV may be appropriate if historical and clinical circumstances are reasonably suggestive of the possibility.

SPECIAL POINTS

Treatment of granuloma annulare depends on the extent of the disease. Localized cases are usually treated with topical or intralesional steroids.

For more widespread cases, phototherapy is often helpful.

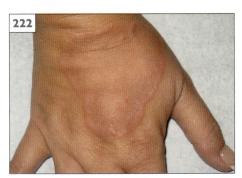

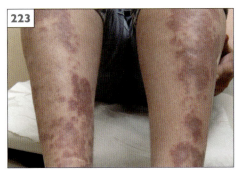

221–223 Granuloma annulare.

Amyloidosis

DEFINITION AND CLINICAL FEATURES

Amyloidosis refers to the abnormal deposition of aggregated proteins in the body. These proteins can exist in the skin in a variety of ways, so amyloidosis of the skin is a diverse condition.

- Primary systemic amyloidosis – is a systemic deposition of amyloid proteins that may involve the skin as well as other organs. External findings include an enlarged tongue (macroglossia), 'pinch purpura' (eccymoses at the sites of minor skin pinching), and waxy pink or yellow papules. Skin findings are not found in up to 60% of patients. This condition affects numerous organs so the patient may have other symptoms as well, including weight loss, fatigue, hoarseness, and hepatomegaly. It may be of idiopathic cause or arise from an underlying plasma cell abnormality, such as multiple myeloma.
- Lichen amyloidosis – is seen at the sites of chronic rubbing or scratching, often on the shins or feet. It usually presents as a rough, 'cobblestone' appearance of flesh-colored or pink papules packed together (**224**). Lichen amyloidosis is thought to arise from cellular contents being repeatedly released from chronic rubbing or scratching.
- Macular amyloidosis – produces itching (sometimes intense) and a grey or dark patch, usually on the upper back. It can be very difficult to treat.
- Primary cutaneous amyloidosis (sometimes called nodular localized amyloidosis) – is rarer and poorly understood. It presents as a single or few firm brown–pink papules at one site on the body. It does not usually itch (**225**).

EPIDEMIOLOGY

Primary amyloidosis is rare in general but more common in the elderly, who can be more prone to underlying conditions such as multiple myeloma. The mean age of onset is 65.

Lichen amyloidosis is uncommon and seen most frequently in middle-aged and older patients.

Macular amyloidosis is relatively common and seen in adults. It is more common in persons of Asian or Middle Eastern descent.

Primary cutaneous amyloidosis is quite rare and seems to be a condition of adults, with a mean age of onset of 55.

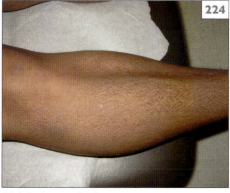

224 Lichen amyloidosis.

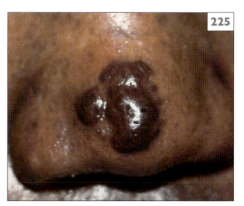

225 Primary cutaneous (nodular) amyloidosis.

DIFFERENTIAL DIAGNOSIS AND INVESTIGATIONS

The differential diagnosis depends on the type of amyloidosis considered. For primary amyloidosis, pinch purpura may be mimicked by senile purpura, anticoagulant medications, or clotting/platelet abnormalities. It is an important condition to diagnose, since it has many systemic manifestations. Skin biopsy is helpful if positive, but cannot exclude the diagnosis. Fat aspiration or rectal biopsy has a higher yield but is more difficult to perform. Serum and urine protein electrophoresis studies can detect abnormal proteins.

Lichen amyloidosis is usually diagnosed based on a history of chronic scratching and the characteristic clinical findings. It may, however, potentially mimic other dermal diseases such as sarcoidosis or pretibial myxedema. A biopsy is definitive and can be stained with Congo red to highlight the amyloid proteins.

Macular amyloidosis is usually distinctive clinically, although it may mimic other itchy dermatoses such as eczema. A biopsy will demonstrate amyloid deposits in the dermal papillae.

Primary cutaneous amyloidosis is often confused with other dermal papules or nodules including sarcoidosis, colloid milium, or cutaneous lymphoma. Biopsy should reveal amyloid as well as plasma cells.

SPECIAL POINTS

The treatment of primary systemic amyloidosis is complex and requires workup for underlying plasma cell dyscrasias. If the diagnosis is suspect based on skin findings, the patient's primary care physician and an experienced oncologist should be involved.

Lichen amyloidosis can be difficult to treat as extensive damage to the skin has usually already been done by the time of diagnosis. Certainly the patient should be encouraged to avoid rubbing or scratching the skin and should avoid using any items or devices to scratch. Potent topical steroids (such as clobetasol ointment) under occlusion with plastic wrap may be helpful. Antihistamines can also be helpful but the more sedating types (such as hydroxyzine and doxepin), which are most helpful for itching, may cause confusion or falls in elderly patients. Intralesional steroids may also work for specific lesions or areas.

Macular amyloidosis is notoriously difficult to treat; the goal should be to reduce or avoid scratching. Topical or intralesional steroids are sometimes helpful. Sedating antihistamines can decrease itching, but must be used with caution in elderly patients. Topical capsaicin is useful if used repeatedly for several weeks or months. It can sting or burn when applied and can cause dramatic pain if spread to the eyes, so patients should wash their hands after applying it.

Treatment of primary cutaneous amyloidosis centers around removing or destroying the nodule. Numerous methods, including surgical excision, curettage, cryotherapy, and ablative lasers, have been used.

Stasis dermatitis

DEFINITION AND CLINICAL FEATURES

Stasis dermatitis is an eczematous skin disorder that occurs on the lower extremities of patients with chronic venous insufficiency. The condition is typically bilateral, although it may be more severe in one leg. The condition results in eczematous, weeping, and scaling plaques overlying pitting edema of the distal lower extremities (**226**). Pruritus is often intense. Venous hypertension leads to extravasation of red blood cells into the tissues with resultant red-brown discoloration of the skin second to hemosiderin deposition. If frank ulceration develops, it is more likely to involve the watershed area of the medial ankle.

It is well recognized that patients with stasis dermatitis more often develop allergic contact dermatitis. This may be a multifactorial process, as patients with stasis dermatitis often use multiple topical medicaments, but also the preexisting dermatitis leads to skin breakdown and may leave one predisposed to the development of a hypersensitivity response.

EPIDEMIOLOGY

Stasis dermatitis is quite common in the elderly population, but it rarely occurs before the fifth decade of life, unless there are other reasons for the patient to manifest acquired venous insufficiency, such as prior surgery, trauma, or thrombosis. The prevalence of stasis dermatitis is estimated to be about 6–7% in patients >50 years of age; when considering only persons >70 years of age, the prevalence of stasis dermatitis may exceed 20%.

Stasis dermatitis is often the earliest manifestation of venous insufficiency, and many affected patients have congestive heart failure and other related conditions. It may also be a harbinger to more problematic conditions yet to foment, such as venous leg ulceration and even lipodermatosclerosis (**227**).

DIFFERENTIAL DIAGNOSIS AND INVESTIGATIONS

The differential diagnosis of stasis dermatitis includes other eczematous conditions (such as nummular dermatitis, contact dermatitis, and so on) as well as other superficial non-melanoma skin cancers. Tinea enters the differential diagnosis as well, and a KOH preparation for microscopic examination may be useful in this regard.

As there are no histological findings that are pathognomonic for stasis dermatitis, a skin biopsy generally shows only non-specific features of eczema, but the test may be useful in excluding other neoplastic processes and tinea.

All patients with stasis dermatitis deserve a complete history and physical examination to assess for the possibility of congestive heart failure, renal failure, or other reasons for volume overload and venous hypertension. Laboratory testing should be guided by the history and physical exam.

SPECIAL POINTS

Patients with stasis dermatitis can help prevent flares by elevating the legs when at rest and wearing compression hosiery when up and about. Gentle bathing and daily application of moisturizer should be recommended. Consultation with a vascular surgeon may be helpful if severe or painful varicosities are present. If severe edema is present, medical management with diuretics will often be helpful.

When the dermatitis is active, a mid-potency topical steroid (such as triamcinolone ointment) is often helpful as needed.

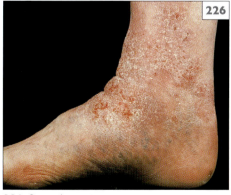

226 Stasis dermatitis.

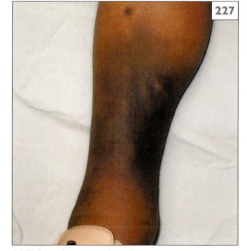

227 Lipodermatosclerosis.

Leg ulcers

DEFINITION AND CLINICAL FEATURES

Leg ulcers are a common problem in elderly patients and have many potential causes. It is important to investigate possible underlying factors, since leg ulcers may be the presenting symptoms of potentially dangerous systemic conditions. The lower leg can be one of the poorest healing areas of the body owing to its dependent position and less effective circulation.

An ulcer is defined as full-thickness loss of the epidermis. The surrounding skin may or may not be normal based on the underlying condition. These include:

- Traumatic – a common cause of ulcers, which can usually be discerned via history, but in elderly patients with altered mental status it may be more difficult. Traumatic ulcers usually have linear, sharply defined edges and should heal with time if treated properly. It is important to watch for secondary infection.
- Infectious – ulcers may be caused by a variety of infections, including common *Staphylococcus aureus* and other bacteria. More unusual fungi (such as *Sporotrichosis* or *Cryptococcus*) or atypical mycobacteria (such as Buruli ulcer caused by *Mycobacterium ulcerans*) are also potential causes. Common skin dermatophyte fungi do not cause ulcers. Infectious ulcers may exhibit drainage or pus and can be difficult to diagnose, so swab and tissue cultures are often needed (**228**).
- Neoplastic – non-melanoma skin cancers, especially squamous cell carcinoma, are a commonly missed cause of leg ulcers.

Neoplastic ulcers may feature adjacent signs of more typical squamous cell carcinoma including scaly nodules or induration. It is important to biopsy any chronic, non-healing ulcer to rule out this possibility.

- Diabetic – one of the most common causes of ulceration is underlying diabetes. In diabetics there is often diminished circulatory effectiveness, neuropathy leading to undetected trauma, and increased risk of infection, all of which can contribute to ulceration. If not treated, these ulcers can easily become infected and lead to amputation. Any elderly patient with a non-healing ulcer should undergo testing for diabetes.
- Vascular – ulceration from insufficient circulatory function is common in the elderly. Arterial ulcers tend to be on the dorsum of the foot or ankle and are usually quite painful (**229**). Venous ulcers are the most common cause of leg ulcers and can affect the entire lower leg with the medial lower leg most common (**230**). They are usually shallower and less painful than arterial ulcers. Signs of underlying stasis dermatitis may be present.

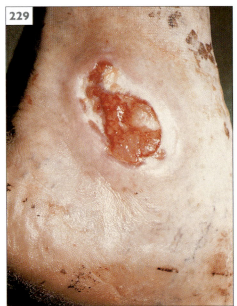

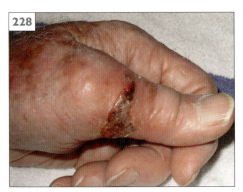

228 Infectious ulcer due to *nocardia*.

229 Arterial ulcer.

- Pressure sores – often seen in elderly and immobile patients. They overlie pressure points such as the sacrum or ankles and arise from chronic pressure. They often become secondarily infected.
- Chronic diseases – certain more unusual systemic diseases, such as pyoderma gangrenosum, pancreatic cancer, ulcerative colitis, and Crohn disease, may be associated with skin manifestations and ulceration.

EPIDEMIOLOGY

Leg ulcers may occur in any age group but are extremely common in the elderly. Patients with poor general health or underlying medical conditions are more prone to many forms of leg ulcers.

DIFFERENTIAL DIAGNOSIS AND INVESTIGATIONS

A thorough history and physical examination are critical in elderly patients with leg ulcer, as there are many (and potentially overlapping) causes. Basic assessment of the circulatory system via examination of distal pulses, capillary refill, edema, and the overlying skin is an important place to start. Further testing should be based on clinical suspicion.

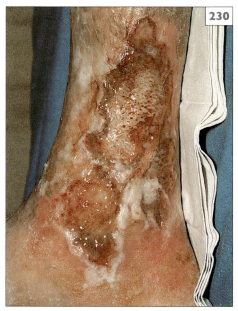

230 Venous (or varicose) ulcer.

Testing for common underlying conditions, including blood glucose levels and an ultrasound of the legs, is often helpful. Wounds that do not heal despite treatment may need cultures to exclude primary or secondary infection and biopsy to exclude skin cancers. It is important to pursue the diagnosis, since treatment is largely based on the underlying cause.

SPECIAL POINTS

Basic treatment of leg ulcers includes gently cleaning the wound and applying an appropriate dressing. Many topical treatments and dressings are available based on the type and size of the wound. Consultation with a specialist wound care provider may be helpful in chronic wound management.

For venous ulcers, elevation and compression are often very helpful. Treating edema medically with diuretics may also help. Vigorous monitoring for and treatment of infection are required. Consultation with a vascular surgeon may be helpful if treatable underlying venous conditions exist.

Diabetics should be advised about the potential for leg ulcers and should see their physician immediately if one occurs. Again, elevation and compression may be helpful. They should clean their feet fastidiously every day, wear clean socks daily, shake out the shoes prior to wearing, and monitor visually for minor injuries which may not be felt due to neuropathy.

It is critical to keep an open mind about potential causes of leg ulceration, especially when an ulcer is not healing as expected. Infectious, malignant, or systemic causes of ulceration require aggressive treatment of the underlying condition to improve.

Leukocytoclastic vasculitis
(hypersensitivity vasculitis)

DEFINITION AND CLINICAL FEATURES
Leukocytoclastic vasculitis (LCV), also known as hypersensitivity vasculitis, is a reactive condition characterized by the deposition of immune complexes in the post-capillary venule, with resultant acute inflammation leading to the classic, non-blanching, raised, 'palpable purpura' (**231–233**). Associated physical findings may include minor joint swelling and arthralgias. The disease is most common on the lower extremities, due to more sluggish blood flow, but in severe cases, it can occur on the upper extremities or even the trunk.

EPIDEMIOLOGY
LCV may occur in any age group. In children, the condition is most often related to infection with *Streptococcus* elsewhere in the body. In adults, it may still be due to *Streptococcus*, or it may be a reaction pattern to other infections (including hepatitis C), medications, connective tissue disease, or a host of other conditions.

Because of the number of elderly persons with polypharmacy, a thorough review of medications started near to the development of the eruption is always indicated. In truth, many series have shown that the cause of LCV in any particular individual is not typically identified.

DIFFERENTIAL DIAGNOSIS AND INVESTIGATIONS
When true palpable purpura is present, LCV is at the top of the differential diagnosis. Disseminated intravascular coagulation can lead to the cutaneous manifestation, purpura fulminans, but this is not usually a palpable purpura and is more macular. Basic histology in LCV will demonstrate a small vessel vasculitis with leukocytoclasia.

Henoch–Schönlein purpura is related to LCV, but it is caused by the deposition of IgA-based complexes, and is associated with gastrointestinal distress, nephritis, and hematuria. Direct immunofluorescence studies are useful in evaluating for Henoch–Schönlein purpura.

A thorough review and physical exam is requisite to identifying any underlying infec-

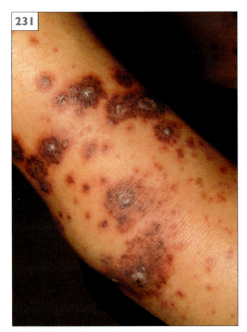

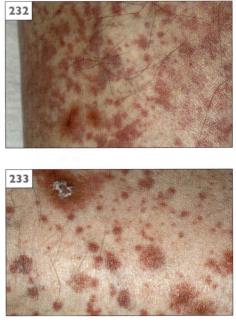

231–233 Leukocytoclastic vasculitis.

tious process in cases of LCV. Urinalysis for hematuria, and blood tests for possible systemic vasculitis (such as ESR and creatinine), are prudent whenever there is even minimal suspicion of nephritis or hematuria.

SPECIAL POINTS

Determining and treating the underlying cause (where possible) is the first step in treating LCV. As with stasis dermatitis, elevation of the legs and compression stockings may be helpful.

For idiopathic cases, topical steroids may be used where mild and systemic steroids for more severe cases. Longer-term treatment can be accomplished with antineutrophil agents, such as colchicine and dapsone, where needed.

Xanthomas

DEFINITION AND CLINICAL FEATURES

Xanthomas are characterized by accumulations of lipid material and/or lipid-laden macrophages within the skin. Sometimes xanthomas can be a reflection of alterations in normal lipid metabolism or they may be idiopathic. Often the clinical manifestations and presentation of the disease are impacted by the type of hyperlipidemia involved. The types of xanthomas that will be briefly outlined include:

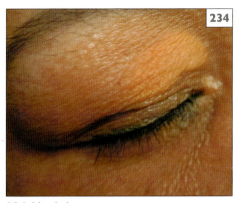

234 Xanthelasma.

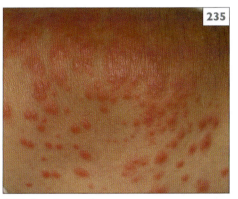

235 Eruptive xanthoma.

- Xanthelasma – asymptomatic and usually bilateral and symmetric accumulations of lipid leading to soft, velvety, yellow, flat papules and small plaques around the eyelids (**234**). Only about one-half of instances of xanthelasma are associated with a recognized lipid abnormality, meaning that testing will often demonstrate no lipid abnormality at all.
- Eruptive xanthomas – rapidly evolving crops of small, red–yellow papules on an erythematous base which often occur on the buttocks, shoulders, and extensor surfaces of the extremities (**235**). Pruritus is common. Eruptive xanthomas are associated with hypertriglyceridemia and they often occur in association with new-onset diabetes.
- Tuberous/tendinous xanthomas – firm, painless, red–yellow nodules that typically develop over the knees, elbows (**236**), and buttocks, or, in the case of tendinous xanthomas, over a tendon (such as the Achilles). Tuberous and tendinous

236 Tuberous/ tendinous xanthoma.

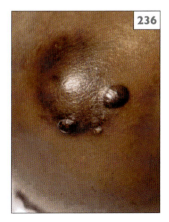

xanthomas are particularly associated with hypercholesterolemia and increased levels of LDL, and they may occur in familial dysbetalipoproteinemia and familial hypercholesterolemia.

- Planar xanthomas – planar xanthomas are nearly completely flat (macular) and rarely form elevated lesions. Generalized planar xanthomas can cover large areas of the face, neck, thorax, and flexural areas. They are sometimes associated with multiple myeloma.

EPIDEMIOLOGY

To a large degree, the prevalence of xanthomas depends on the prevalence of the underlying lipid abnormalities, which is beyond the scope of this discussion. Suffice to say that xanthomas may occur at any age, although xanthelasma in particular is most common in persons >50 years old.

DIFFERENTIAL DIAGNOSIS AND INVESTIGATIONS

Eruptive xanthomas can be confused with other pruritic inflammatory conditions such as dermatitis herpetiformis. Tuberous and tendinous xanthomas may be confused with cutaneous cysts and lipomas. Skin biopsy will confirm the diagnosis, and, on discovery of xanthomas, studies to rule out hyperlipidemia are appropriate. Serum levels of triglycerides and cholesterol should be measured following a 12-hour fast. In the case of planar xanthoma, a serum and urine protein electrophoresis is also indicated.

SPECIAL POINTS

It is important to determine the type of xanthoma present to detect and treat any underlying lipid abnormality. Xanthoma associated with elevated lipids may improve as the lipids normalize. Excisional surgery or destruction of individual lesions may be helpful, although recurrence is common.

Erythema gyratum repens

DEFINITION AND CLINICAL FEATURES

Erythema gyratum repens (EGR) is a paraneoplastic figurate (reactive) erythema that forms characteristic concentric erythematous bands with a 'wood-grain appearance.' There is a rapid migratory and changing quality to the pattern of scaling on the body. The eruption is pruritic.

The pathogenesis of this disorder is poorly understood, but it is suspected that tumor antigens cross-react with endogenous skin antigens and/or tumor cells, or invading inflammatory cells elaborate cytokines, perpetuating the inflammation and stimulating keratinocytes and other normal cellular constituents of the skin.

The condition is associated with malignancy in at least 80% of patients and so, although rare overall, it favors elderly patients. Lung cancer is most often associated with the disease, although it has also been identified in association with cancer of the breast, bladder, uterus/cervix, and stomach. Usually the development of the eruption precedes other symptoms of the cancer.

EPIDEMIOLOGY

EGR is a very rare condition with thorough reviews identifying only about 50 patients within the literature. Most of these cases were reported in white people. Typically the condition presents in persons >40 years of age, with a mean age of 63 years, and males are affected twice as often as females.

DIFFERENTIAL DIAGNOSIS AND INVESTIGATIONS

Other reactive and figurate erythemas, such as erythema annulare centrifugum, may be confused with EGR. The scaling and migratory quality of the annular lesions may also mimic tinea infection. In this regard, a KOH examination and skin biopsy may be useful in excluding other conditions and suggesting the diagnosis, although the histological findings of EGR are not specific. Studies to identify any associated malignancy should be based on the patient's age and the impression and results from a thorough history and physical examination.

SPECIAL POINTS

As with other paraneoplastic skin conditions, treatment of EGR involves detecting and treating the underlying malignancy. The skin condition may resolve with successful treatment of the cancer, where possible.

Acrokeratosis neoplastica
(Bazex syndrome)

DEFINITION AND CLINICAL FEATURES
Acrokeratosis neoplastica, also known as Bazex syndrome, is a rare paraneoplastic condition most often associated with squamous cell carcinoma of the upper aerodigestive tract. It is rare in general, but when found is often in older patients.

The condition manifests as symmetric, scaling erythematous to slightly violaceous plaques on the hands and fingers (**237**). The condition may also affect the feet, nose, and helices of the ears.

EPIDEMIOLOGY
Only about 140 cases are reported in the literature, and in these cases males greatly outnumbered females by a ratio of about 12:1. In one particular review, the mean age of onset was 61 years. Both of these epidemiological observations are impacted by the increased prevalence of squamous cell carcinoma of the aerodigestive tract in elderly individuals and, in particular, in males.

DIFFERENTIAL DIAGNOSIS AND INVESTIGATIONS
Bazex syndrome can be confused with psoriasis, chronic hand dermatitis, and other eczematous conditions. Unlike these other conditions, and considering the paraneoplastic nature of the condition, Bazex syndrome is often distinguished by a recalcitrant course in comparison to these other diseases.

A skin biopsy is indicated, as is a KOH examination to exclude tinea. While the histological findings of Bazex syndrome are not specific, the value of the biopsy lies in the ability to exclude other conditions. A thorough history and physical examination is indicated and, based on the findings therein, additional testing modalities to identify the underlying malignancy are appropriate.

SPECIAL POINTS
The key to treatment is detection and treatment of the underlying malignancy. If it can be successfully treated, the skin will often improve. Topical keratolytics (such as urea cream or ammonium lactate lotion) may be helpful symptomatically.

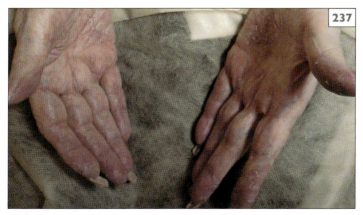

237 Bazex syndrome.